I'm hoping that you will get something out of this, and that it
will help you? Since that's the whole purpose that I've done this,
because it was important to me... To share my own personal
story, and things I've been through. Believing that it could be
useful to others... Who's struggling with having Epilepsy? I
know how it affects you, and what it's like? I hope that you can
have a healing journey, but a remarkable breakthrough with your
Epilepsy, too! Be kind, gentle, and love yourself!!! Be good to
yourself, and do your best.

Sincerely,

Ginger Scott

Chapters: (1-13)

My Journey with Epilepsy & Getting Through It

By

GINGER SCOTT

Chapter 1. The Beginning

My name is Ginger, and I'm 45 years old. I have a problem
that I've struggled with my whole life... Since I was a child, and
I'm an Epileptic; but I also have Non-Epileptic Seizures, too!
I've got 4 kinds of Seizure Disorders, and they are as follows:
Grandma Epileptic Seizures, Partial Onset Seizures, Pseudo
Seizures & Non-Partial Non-Epileptic Seizures, too! That's the
four kinds of seizures that it took my entire life... To finally find
out that I was having? I started having seizures as a baby, but my
family... Didn't think that much of it, because they didn't
believe it was anything to worry about? I slept right through a
Tornado when I was inside my baby crib sleeping, and it had
came right through our neighborhood when I was a child?

I had falls, but also I lost control of my bladder… Due to the seizures, and I didn't have any control over it either! It's not funny, because I know… How embarrassing it is? Plus, it is something that often happens when people suffer with Seizure Disorders. It's not something that you can control, and it's just like when you lose consciousness? You don't have any control over that either do you? No, I don't think so… I heard from others when I was growing up? That I had fallen out of bed multiple times, too!

I didn't know what was happening to me? I didn't know I'd even fallen out of bed? I did know that I woke up on the floor, and didn't know… How I'd gotten onto the floor? I had problems with my speech, and couldn't pronounce words correctly. That lasted all my life, because there's still sometimes that happens… Due to my speech not allowing me to control my words when they come out? Plus, when I'm going to have seizures sometimes that happens, too? It also has happened before & after, them at times. I've been told by others, but I've had many near death experiences; because of my Epilepsy & Seizures, too!

Being so far out of control that they nearly killed me, because my heart stopped beating; and I turned blue in the face! I've been resuscitated a numerous amount of times, because of what happened to me? When I'd had the seizures, and almost died? I also have seen multiple Neurologists, because of my seizures that I've had. It's taken a long time, and a lot of patience… With experimenting with multiple medications that could treat Epilepsy. That would also at the same time cooperate with my body, and me not have an Allergic Reaction to them. Or my seizures worsen, because of the medications? I've had all kinds of scans such as MRI's, CT's, & EEG's done. With & without the video, too!

It's not been a very easy road to travel, and walk down... For a very long time. I wasn't sure? I was even going to make it, because they've been so bad. It took many times of me acting like their guinea pig... In order for them to find what might possibly work? Every time it seemed that sometimes things would work for a little while, but then there'd be more issues. Making it almost feel hopeless, because they would have to try something different again. It was like being at square one all over again, too! Sometimes I had to even deal with the thoughts of suicide, because of the side effects from the medicine; and that was what had caused it?

Sometimes that does happen, but you're warned about it... Anytime they put you on a medicine and combos, together. Since it's something that you have to really pay attention, too! Others inside your life must also be aware... Of any problems, because sometimes you might not see them? Some of the reactions caused by the medications, and you need some help? Getting back to your doctor, because they need to do something else to help you. Or make an adjustment, and see if that works? It's also not fun... Having to have your blood tested all the time, because of levels for the medications.

Since they have to check to make sure that your medication is at the right does, but also that you're body organs... Are functioning properly, too! It's very important that they do follow up with you regularly, and make sure... That everything is ok? Since it's your life that it's concerning, because you're important! I have a scar in my left lobal temporal, and a bruise on the back of my skull. I was also beaten as a child, but it's caused me to have permanent brain damage. That's irreversible, too! It showed up on my tests before, but there's nothing that can be done about it. It'll never go away, and it causes me to feel not like a normal person, too!

Especially since I have the Epilepsy, and it's possible that they could've stopped my seizures... If I hadn't experienced the severe trauma that I did growing up? Epilepsy skipped every 3 generations inside my family on my mom's side, but I wasn't one of the lucky ones? I ended up having it! That doesn't make me feel like I'm lucky at all, but more like I'm cursed. By a disease that'll never disappear! Only I know how precious life is? I also know that it's by the Grace of God... That I'm even alive, because I should've not been here! Since I've had so many near death experiences, but also by what I grew up around... Being inside of such a violent, abusive, childhood home that was dysfunctional as all get out!

I also realize that I'm a very beautiful person from the inside & out, too! That God created me for a reason, and I feel like I've a purpose. I am gifted with Spiritual Gifts, but I also know what they're all about? I am very smart, bright, intelligent, and just like anyone else... Other than the fact, that I'm an Epileptic. That doesn't make you a bad person, and nobody should ever say these words to you: "I wish you were dead! Since all you do? Is have seizures all the time! I hate you, because you're an Epileptic!"

Believe me, I was told that... Along with I was a mistake that never should've happened growing up by people in my family. Do you know what that feels like? Not very good at all! I ended up leaving home, and headed out on my own... I don't regret it, but I also don't recommend doing that. I didn't have anyone to help me, because nobody loved me. Nobody cared about me whether if I died or survived? Except for two people! That was me & God, too!

We were the only ones that really cared, and I made sure that I did my best... Of what I could? To make things better, because I was in a horrible situation that wasn't going to turn out very good. I had lost the other people from my family that did care about me, and that hurt very bad, too! Since they were the only ones who did? I managed, but made good... On my own of taking care of myself the best ways that I could, and made sure. That I did get the help I needed to deal with my problems, too! Not just trying to escape from my childhood home, but also to handle the other problems... My Epilepsy & Health Issues, that I had to deal with.

I didn't just suffer from Epilepsy, but had other seizures to deal with... Along with Post Traumatic Stress Disorder, Severe Major Depression, Abuse Issues to work through also. Plus, I had some problems with my Back, Hands, Legs & Thyroid, too! I also had to deal with some Flashbacks of things that had happened, and learn how to deal with them also? Which wasn't very easy to do! It was a hard road, but I managed the best I could... I kept a Journal, and wrote down inside of it my feelings. Or how I was doing? Plus, how things in life were going? I also saw a Counselor, because I needed, too!

In order for me to be able to learn how to deal and manage, all of my problems? Since things were so difficult, but also helping me to move forward... Instead of going backwards, because of where I'd came from? Being inside of an abusive childhood home, and it can be very devastating, too! Keeping a person wrapped up inside a shell, but also in a dangerous spot. Since they might not always be so willing to reach out to others... When they need it the most? Or if they need any help, and are having a hard time coping with life? There are those times of darkness... That will appear when we least expect it, too?

It's always good to have somebody there inside your life that you can talk, too! Especially when things get that bad, and you need to be reaching out. Instead of staying withdrawn, but inside your safe zone? I know you might not want to admit it... Everyone has those times at one point in their life, and maybe they don't know what to do? When those moments come? Except having support from others always helps... As long as it's someone that you can count on, and you know you can trust. To help you, but also be there for you! Struggling with Epilepsy isn't an easy thing to handle, and it can be very overwhelming sometimes, too!

Having to always deal with it by yourself isn't cool or fun either. It is nice when you have others that help you in dealing with the problems, and can understand? There's lots of people that have the disease, but sometimes there's those who aren't educated that much about it? Making it harder for them to understand what it's like? Or what it's about? Or how it affects an individual? Controlling their life, and taking over... That's pretty much what it often does? Until you can get some help getting on the right medications, and have a doctor that helps you? Sometimes everyone doesn't need to understand, but don't be ashamed or embarrassed; over it.

Especially since it's not your fault, but there's nothing... That you should feel ashamed or embarrassed, over due to having Epilepsy either. It's something that millions of individuals have, and something that doctors... Have learned a lot about through the years. When I was first diagnosed? At the age of 13 years old they didn't have as many options... As they do now, and they didn't have all the information they do now. Not on me, or the disease itself? I'd been having them before 13 is according to what the Neurologist doctor had stated, but nobody else had really known? What was happening to me?

I'm just like everyone that suffers from this disease of Epilepsy, and have my moments… When I'm sweet, but times when I'm not so nice? Sometimes the seizures can make you quiet hateful, and vey difficult to get along with. Other times they might not affect you that way, but your mood may be more stable. With my Epilepsy it varies depending on how bad the seizures were? What kind they are that I'm having? Plus, how many sets of them I had? They make it often hard to function at times, and can make your whole entire body hurt very bad all over! From the twitching, activity of the seizures & episodes themselves, too? Plus, make you lose your appetite, dry mouth, go to the bathroom a bunch; but also cause you to feel very tired & exhausted, too!

They can affect everything in your life, but be a royal pain… To have to learn how to deal with them? Especially when it's looking not so promising? Due to all the things that your doctors have tried? Only nothing seems like it's working? When they have to find something different to help you? That can be not only aggravating & frustrating, but also disappointing & upsetting; extremely to an Epileptic. Epileptic's are a lot more emotional than most people, because of how they're affected from the seizures & episodes? An individual not on the proper medication or dose? Can become very unstable, and have other multiple issues to deal with also!

It can be very tiring, exhausting & depressing… Trying to find the right things to work, too! Especially when there's times? That it's so difficult, because certain types of things don't want to work at all? That makes it more of a struggle, but it's not just about dealing with Epilepsy… It's way much more than that! You've got to find a new way to live, because it's affecting your whole life? That's the hard part, and why it's so terrible? It overpowers your body, and takes away your freedom… In ways others wouldn't imagine, too!

Sometimes you're not allowed to drive a vehicle, go swimming alone, take a bath by yourself; or go for walks alone? Due to the fact, that you might have seizures, and it wouldn't take long? For something tragic to happen to you! That makes things harder for you, but at the same time… It's also protecting you, and keeping you safe! Especially since you need to make sure that nothing bad happens to you also, but nobody else wants that either? Since it's you that they're looking out for? You can drown in less than an inch of water, but that's not just due the seizures. You don't know when you're going to have them for the most part, and they're unpredictable, too? Seizures have a very amazing, but powerful strength; and they can cause you to drown easily!

I know that, too! It doesn't take very much for awful things to happen, and they can occur… Within just a few seconds with those things, too! That's just how it is? I've broken my ribs, blacked my eyes, busted my lips, busted my nose; but also broken toes before over them. I've also fallen on many different occasions from them happening, too! I've had a terrible time with finding things to help me, and it's been a very unpleasant adventure. Except I'm glad that I'm where I'm today with them also? Since I'm improving, because my doctor has been able to find the right combination of Epileptic Seizure Medications… For me to take, too!

One of my medications had to be completely maxed out at the highest dose possible, but it's working. Then I have another one that was added, too! It is helping me also, but there's lots of side effects, and it's hard getting used to them. Sometimes you never do! It's the complication in my life, and it's always been the biggest problem for me to handle. Since I used to have so many seizures, but had up to 100 a day before… Having back to back sets, and they lasted for very long time periods, too! They ended up causing me to have a Heart Problem, but that is being monitored also. Which is helping me, and there's things in my body… That make me feel like will never get better, because of how bad my seizures were my entire life?

I've got a tongue that looks like a Lizard, because I bit it almost in half! During my seizure episodes, but nobody ever did anything to try to stitch it up? So, it might not have been that bad… If they had? It's split, because of the severity of my seizure activity; and me biting it… With my teeth when I had my Epileptic Seizures, too? It's something that often can happen, too! Seizures are very strong, powerful, and can-do things… That you might not think. Like cause someone to bite a spoon, and swallow it… Or bite of a finger?

If you put something in between their mouth & teeth, during them? You shouldn't do that, because they could choke or hurt themselves & someone else, too! It's not really funny at all… What a person with Epilepsy & Seizures, goes through. I've been made fun of over them before, and I also know. How much that hurts, but how painful it can be, too? Plus, how cruel & insensitive, other people can be? That's when sometimes you've got to learn? How to laugh at yourself? You're not laughing with them, but you're not letting them get to you either!

It's something not only that you learn to live with, but you learn how to handle? Or it'll control you the rest of your life, too? Plus, you learn how to cope with it also, but that does take time… It's not something that happens overnight, and can be very difficult also. The main thing is when you do? How you cope? To deal with the problem, and what's happening to you? Plus, how it's affecting your life also? It also has a really good way of affecting other people's lives… That's inside your life, too!

Since it affects everyone, and not just yourself! It affects everyone around you, but that has a part in your life, too! Sometimes you might tend to forget that, but it also has a way… Of affecting your memory a great deal, and your concentration also. Plus, it can affect your brain, but make it not work properly… You wouldn't think the way you do? Any other time when you're having the seizures? Or after your episodes? You might be very confused, unaware, or unalert? About certain things that you normally would be paying more attention, too!

It causes things to be a lot different than what a person? Who has a normal life has? Things just aren't the same at all, and are more difficult also. Not just for you, but others that play an important part in your life, too! Since it takes more than one person sometimes… To handle such a situation as this. I was going to Speech Therapy. Until I was five years old, because of the difficulty I had talking from my seizure problems? Then I was taken out of regular school, because of them… Being put in a Special School for children who couldn't function inside of a regular school setting?

Due to my Epilepsy, and I missed out on some classes even there. Along with other events that would take place during the school day or activities? Since my teacher's would have to put me inside a room… Where I could rest, because I'd had a bunch of seizures? Plus, I'd thrown up, and they cleaned me up. Also, they had somebody watch me, because they needed to make sure… I was going to be ok? Sometimes an Ambulance was called, because I'd stopped breathing, and my heart stopped, too! I wasn't looked down on here at this school, because other people understood. Since it was a school where a lot of students went with multiple problems, and it wasn't a full day of school either?

Since I wasn't able to handle a full regular school day, because of my Epilepsy & Seizures, I was having all the time. My seizures were out of control for a very long time, too! They were happening more frequently than what everyone wanted them to occur? Except the doctors were having trouble getting things to cooperate… With medications & my body, too! Since my body wasn't accepting a lot of the medications, but having many bad, terrible reactions to them. Causing them not to work, or causing my seizures to worsen also. It was rather embarrassing to me… That I would often lose control of my bladder over having seizures, and didn't have any control over that happening. I had to often take a lot more showers, because of that except I didn't mind cleaning up, but did mind what had just happened?

I never got used to the fact… That I was going to have to depend on others to help me with my problems either, and I didn't like it! It made me angry, aggravated, sad & depressed. Since I wanted to just be able to take care of myself. I also didn't have as much independence sometimes as I wanted? That really frustrated me, too! Since I was pretty independent, and didn't like depending on others that much. I liked taking care of myself, and wasn't happy about that at all. There was lots of things I couldn't do, because of my seizures… That interfered with my daily life, too! That really bothered me, too!

Other's didn't always understand, but picked on me… Due to not being able to understand. What I was going through, and what I was having to deal with all the time? It's not easy being an Epileptic, and having to go through all the problems… That it causes, but also dealing with the consequences. Of the aftereffects of seizures, too! What they do to you, and your body… After you've had them? It's also hard to find the right doctor sometimes, and can take lots of time in doing that, too! It's also a struggle getting up, but getting started on any activities that is right in front of you; because it can have such an impact on your life, mood, motivation & capabilities, to get things finished.

I thought about Suicide a lot, because of not knowing… If I was going to ever stop having seizures? Or them getting better at all? If the doctors were ever going to be able to help me? Or if they'd just give up on me? Well as I got older… They did give up on me, but I found some different doctors. That didn't say it wasn't impossible to help me? They said, it was my medications… That I needed a different combination of medications to help me.

I would feel better, and it was going to take time. We'd have to try some medications that I'd been on before, but that they'd believed I was allergic, too! Except I wasn't allergic to those medications, but it's working! Before all that had happened? I had been put on some medication… That I didn't need to be on at all, and it was an Anti-depressant. I got very depressed, and I took an overdose of all my Seizure Medications & Anti-depressant, too! I was engaged to be married, but ended up being admitted into ICU in a Semi-Coma State, because of trying to kill myself. I was in the hospital for two weeks, and released right before Easter Sunday. I returned home, but had a better Neurologist afterwards; and got a better Counselor to help me with all my problems in life, too!

Boy! Did I really need that, too! She worked with people who had multiple issues, and had been through the kinds of abuse I had been. She only worked with Women, Men & Children, who had been abused in similar ways… That I had been? She was great! She got me right on track, and I had my head on straight afterwards. It took a lot of work, and working through a lot of pain, too! I made it through to the other side, but it was worth every bit of it also. If it hadn't been for her helping me get through all my issues?

I probably wouldn't have married my Spouse, because things were that bad with me. When I had tried to kill myself? I didn't really want to die! That's only how I really felt deep down inside, but not what I really wanted? I almost succeeded in that, too! I'm glad that my fiancé had gotten out of work early, and he found me… He saved my life, but he wasn't the only one. The Paramedics, Rescue Squad, Doctors, Nurses & God, did, too! If it hadn't been for everyone than I might not have survived? I was very confused, and I was upset… I was depressed, sad, and not talking to anyone about how I felt?

Or what was going on with me? That was definitely not the right thing to do! My seizures still remained very bad for a while, but it wasn't long… That they did start improving, too! After getting married? We moved to a different State, and we found some other doctors. It took longer than we expected, because we had to change them a few times… Before we could get me into a better Neurologist, and they be able to help me? That's exactly what they did? I was recommended for Surgery, and it wasn't a simple surgery; but a very dangerous surgery that was considered a special surgery.

I was told that they had a device that was an Implant, but it is just for Epilepsy. It's called a VNS short for Vagus Nerve Stimulator Pulse Generator. I had surgery, and my first one implanted in 2,010. It was the biggest mistake I'd made! I went to surgery early that morning, and I had a great doctor that performed my surgery… Thankfully, I am really glad he was so wonderful! I was put all the way out, but had my chest & neck, cut open… They inserted a device that's metal made like a Pacemaker, but doesn't work the same way inside of my chest. The wire goes up from that piece, and up to my neck; but up by my juggler vein. Then it goes further up towards my brain, and it works 24-7, too!

It's controlled by a device that your doctor has that's a computer wizard tool, but checks the settings. Can increase the settings, or decrease them? Plus, it checks the battery life, too! It can check to see if there's a malfunction, too! Except sometimes the malfunction might not show up on the computer wizard tool the doctor has? I was given medications while under, and had been put on a ventilator. I also died! I saw God, and went up to heaven… Jesus spoke to me, but he told me that he wasn't ready for me to come home yet? He still had something left for me to do on Earth, and he wasn't going to let me die yet?

It wasn't my time! I remember not being able to see his face, but I could see... A bright light, and it was white. Plus, there was a gold Aurora over his head. The sky was so beautiful, and blue... With some flowers everywhere, and there was animals that were everywhere, too! Plus, he let me see... My grandpa, grandma, Mentor & my godparent's, too! That had passed a while back, and that was cool. Was what I thought?

Since I could see those people, and knew exactly where they were at? He sent me back, and I remember this long like tunnel... That I passed through, but then I was looking at my body over the operating table. Before I entered back inside of it, too! That was freaky! I went to the Recovery Room after my surgery, but I was inside surgery a lot longer... Than what I was supposed to be, too? It was supposed to only take an hour and a half, but I was inside of surgery for almost 6 hours. I recovered inside the room that they'd taken me, too! Then they took me back upstairs after I had woken up a little, bit wheeling me into a hospital room.

I was seen by some nurses, and had my vital signs taken... For a little bit, but also they managed my pain. I didn't have any stitches on my neck & throat, but staples. With glue that the doctor had to slap on me... In order to keep me from bleeding to death! Since there could be a lot of blood loss from this kind of procedure, because of how they had to cut you? In order to place the device inside safely? The device is supposed to be turned on in a few weeks after your surgery? As long as you're healing ok, but I wasn't... I had to have my shoulder put back into place, too!

When I went to see the doctor afterwards? I also had some stitches in my chest that were trying to come out... To soon, too! I wasn't healed yet though? I was healing very slowly, but as time went on... I started doing better with my healing. The device hurt when it was turned on, because it made a piercing, sharp, pain inside my chest hurt; but it also shocked my heart. It sent a stimulate shock up to the wire, and was supposed to try to stop or prevent me from having seizures. Except that's not what it did? Plus, it was causing my seizures to become worse, but it seemed like it wasn't working right at all?

It wasn't either, and when I went to Concerts? It interfered with my device. I got shocked by lots of Electrical Appliances at home, because of my device. I was choking a lot, too! I would get the hiccups from the device, and I got strangled often... Due to choking from the stimulation of the device. I also got burned from some things, too! My heart stopped a whole bunch of times, too! It was happening a lot, too! I suffered a lot of harm, because of having the device put inside of my body?

I have some permanent damage caused by the VNS device, and regret that I ever had them put inside of me. My whole goal was to get better, but not end up with more problems. That didn't happen with the VNS device, and I had 2 put inside of my body. The battery didn't last the lifespan it was supposed, too! My first implant lasted for two years, and that was it. My second one malfunctioned, and I went into seizures... That almost caused me to not come out, but almost died. I don't remember even going to the hospital inside of an Ambulance or calling 911! My Spouse told me what had happened? I had no idea!

They decided inside the hospital to shut off the device, and recommended that it stay placed inside of my body. That it was too dangerous to try to remove, because of the seriousness of my condition. Plus, the seriousness of the problems that could arise during surgery... If they tried to remove the entire device? Except they couldn't remove all of it anyway, because they have to leave a small part of the wire inside of you... Since it can be entirely removed. After it was shutoff? I had seizures that were very bad, but caused me to break the device... I guess that doesn't really matter much though, because nobody's doing anything with it anyway. Except I was told they weren't supposed to leave it inside of you, and not broken either?

It doesn't matter from what my new doctor says? That makes me feel better, and he doesn't recommend them being used either. That made me feel better, too! Since I feel like they're very bad, too! They do cause lots of problems, and I also fell a lot with my devices, too! My Spouse had to pick me up out of the floor lots of times, because of that. He believes that treating them with medications are better, but not those kinds of devices. I agree, but sometimes that is difficult. After learning what I have now? I regret ever having it done?

My doctor told me that it's not going to cause a problem just leaving it there. Since it's broken, but off, too! They know it's broken, because it won't even register now at all. That's how they know, but don't know... Where it's broken at? It could be broken on the metal part that's inside my chest. Or the wire could be broken? Or they both could be broken, too? Nobody knows for sure. There's only one way for them to find out? That's by surgery, and that's not happening!

Chapter 2. Coping

How've I learned how to cope with all of this you might be asking? Well it's not been very easy, but I've found my own ways. One way that I learned how to cope with this was by counseling, and another was by journaling. Also, I've learned how to use music? To help me cope & heal, but handle all my problems. Giving all my problems to God, and letting him handle them. Plus, by writing, drawing, creativity & singing. Plus, by enjoying things that I couldn't enjoy before in life… Going to do things for fun when I can? Working on myself, and building my self-esteem… Plus, being able to relax by enjoying video games occasionally, and relaxing with them.

They help me destress sometimes, too! Trying to take care of myself the best way that I can. No matter if it means that I need more sleep than others sometimes, but can function maybe at opposite hours. Than your average person? Plus, keeping myself in tabs with what's going on with me? Making sure that I have everything in check with myself, and how I'm feeling? Plus, trying to make sure that I do everything within my power… That I can to keep myself in good shape, too! Which isn't as easy as it used to be? Since I've a lot more problems to deal with, but I do try.

Finding love in my pets, nature, music & the little things in life… That make me happy, too! Plus, enjoying spending time with my Spouse. Making sure that I keep all my appointments if possible? When I need to go back to see my doctors again? Since I've multiple doctors, because of all my problems that I've got. That's very important, too! I had to process everything that had happened? When I had attempted suicide back in 2,004? That was really hard getting through all of it, but I was successful in doing so.

I had a lot of support from my friends, counselor, Fiancé & doctors, too. Plus, being able to use God anytime to talk, too! When I didn't feel like I could to anyone else… That really helped me a lot, too! Jesus & I, are very close to each other… I've got him wrapped around my little pinky, and we talk all the time, together. I'm very special he told me, because I'm one of his children… Plus, he's blessed me with all kinds of Spiritual Gifts, and a few Psychic Capabilities, too! Nope, it's not really what you're thinking? I'm not a witch, but I can see things that other people can't.

I can see Spirits, and I've got Discernment & Discerning of the Spirits. What's that mean? Well I can see spirits from the other side. I can see Spirits that are pure from Christ, and I can see Spirits if they're not pure. I can command them, and tell them to leave! If they're not pure from Christ, but of the Devil himself… Plus, I can keep them from hurting others, too! I can send them back to where they came from? If they are from Christ then I usually always allow them to stay, because I know they mean no harm. They are here for a special reason, and sometimes it's; because God has sent them to give me a message. Or to watch over me, but sometimes there's another reason… They want my help with something?

Along with a bunch of other gifts that he's given me, too! Not just the discernment & discerning of spirit's, but he's given me all kinds of Spiritual Gifts… I was tested by a test that the man who was my Mentor? Gave me to take, but he did this before I got married to my Spouse. That doesn't really matter that much, because it's still the same. He was also the man who married up? He knew what he was talking about, too! It's a test that is a Biblical Test, and only a Minister or someone with Bible Teaching & Knowledge, can give this test appropriately. It's a handwritten test, and you answer all the questions. There's two forms a long one, and a short one, too!

I've had so many near death experiences that I honestly believe... God's been watching over me, and protecting me the whole time. As crazy as this might sound... I could hear Angels singing from heaven. Before I was born inside my mother's womb, and it made me feel safer. I could see things... That were happening before I was born, and I believe that's why? I didn't want to come out when I was supposed, too? God gave me a message recently, but it wasn't something I understood at first. It came to me in a dream... When I was sleeping one night, and not feeling very good?

Jesus said, "I'm using you as a tool for all these doctors to learn from you... So, that they can help others, and you're my instrument of peace, love & kindness. For them to learn from, because of all your health problems... Even though this might not seem fair to you, but it's not punishment. You're a good lesson for them to study, but be able to use for future medical conditions... Since you've all the problems you've got, and if they use your body & health, correctly? They can achieve things to help lots of other people, too!"

The reason that he said, this is; because I've multiple complex issues... That some doctors don't know how to handle? Also a lot of them are linked to other problems that I've got, too! Which makes it even more complicated sometimes to see... What's really going on with me? I have some problems that have been caused to worsen, because of other problems. Or to occur from pre-existing conditions, too! I have lots of ways that I've used for coping though... Exercise used to be a really big one, too! I'd go walking a lot, but things got difficulty with my walking; and caused it to become harder for me to do so much of, too!

I love using the music & writing, a lot! It really helps, and since my seizures… Are improved now with the medication combo that I'm taking. I can achieve that a lot more! I still have all the other problems, but Epilepsy isn't my only Neurological problem. I also have other Neurological disorders, and one that I'm aware of is: Peripheral Neuropathy. It's extremely painful, too! It causes a whole lot of pain, but makes my feet actually feel like they're on fire! When I try walking?

The pain radiates, and it causing me all kinds of problems, too! They don't know what caused this? I had my hands & feet, burned when I was a child? I don't know if that caused this to happen later on or not? It's not something that you're born with, but it's terrible trying to deal with! Right now my spouse and I, are wondering? If it's attacking my Auto-Immune System? Since I'm very sick, but having all kinds of issues with my stomach… Plus, severe nausea & vomiting, and I'm not able to eat a lot of things. My body is starting to reject certain foods, beverages & medications, too!

This can happen after the Neuropathy gets to a certain point, and mine hasn't been treated for a long time. I also suffer with having Fibromyalgia, too! With everything combined, together… It's extremely painful & difficult! I try the best I can to manage, but sometimes it's so painful… That it's hard to sleep, or get out of bed. Sometimes it makes me feel so bad… That I stay home a lot, because of how terrible I'm feeling? It isolates me, and controls my life often… Due to how terrible it makes me feel, too?

It doesn't get easier to deal with, and it's not anything that's going away! It's here to stay, but along with the rest of my problems, too! It's very frustrating & aggravating, but lots of sleepless times... Due to the problems, too! Plus, there's times when I'll sleep too much, because of lack of sleep? Since it's made me feel so bad? I'm glad that I have a Spouse who does understand... What I'm going through? He's been on my side more than anybody else had at all during the whole time... He's watched me suffering with all my problems, and more than most of my doctors, too!

There's been a concern about me getting Lupus, too! From me having all the Neurological problems... That's already existing, too! From one of my previous Neurological doctors, and I really hope that doesn't happen... If it does? My Spouse said, "We'll deal with it step by step... One thing at a time, but that's not very comforting." Even though I do know what he means, but it's just depressing... Knowing that could happen, too! That same doctor was concerned about my body shutting down at some point, and rejecting medications & food, too!

This has been happening to me for months now, and we've had to experiment with what I can eat if anything sometimes? He was also concerned about other Neurological disorders coming up, too! He said, "It didn't mean they would? Except that's always possible with Epileptics, because of everyone being different; and their health complications? He wasn't sure if it was going to happen, but was afraid about it doing that with me?" Since I kept having more & more, problems that would keep occurring... Making it very difficult for them to treat me, too! Some issues can come from other problems, and be linked right back to other problems that already exist. It's not been easy trying to handle all these problems, but I feel blessed... Instead of feeling bad about myself, because I know God is watching over me.

That things could always be worse, too! I currently don't have Lupus, but there's still a lot of things happening to me & my body; that we don't understand? That are causing some major issues, and making things really hard for me, too! That doesn't mean that it's not something that can't happen, because we were told... That it sure could, too! That does worry me, too! Except I know that worrying about it isn't going to do any good... So, I just have to keep my chin up, and move on forward. Keep putting one foot in front of the other one, but not give up doing what I want to do? What is it that I want to do?

I want to continue being an Author! That's what I want to do, and what I planned on doing before? Except that was put on hold for a little while, because of my seizures... Being so far out of control. That I was unable to go forward, but also they caused me a Heart Problem, and we had to deal with that, too! That was very challenging, but I'm stable... Taking daily medications, and they're required to keep me alive! Without them I could die? They are life savers for me, and so is Jesus, too! Without him I'd be nothing?

It's taken a long time to get me in under someone's care, and get me... To the point at where I'm at today? My previous doctor started it, and he was Dr. Rodney Quinn. When we moved away? My new doctor finished up what he started? Adding a different medication, but starting me out slowly... Which you have to always do? Then gradually increasing the medication as you go. So, one of my Epileptic Medications is maxed out, because they didn't have a choice! Except to increase the dose to the highest dose, because my body needed it.

Along with the second medication, too! It's working, and I'm on 3,000 mg. of Keppra every day. Along with 750 mg. of Depakote every day, too! That's what's made me become more stable though. Plus, getting my other medications that I needed at the right doses, too! Plus, making sure that I have routine labs… Along with seeing my doctor when I need, too? I have more needs than some people, but I'm glad… That there's people who are there to help me, and are taking care of me the way I need, too! It's working for me though, ant that's the most important thing, too!

I'm really grateful for my doctors helping me, and the ones who have? They all know who they are, too? Especially since it's not always that easy, but I can't say thanks enough… To all of them, because I'm really glad that they were there for me. To help me, too! Without everyone's help, and the love & support… That my spouse has given to me. Being right beside my side, and not giving up; but trying his best to get through all this with me. I'm really glad that I have such a wonderful man, who understood; but seen first-hand… What it was like?

For me, and could tell my doctors what I couldn't, because I had no idea… About some of the things he had to tell them for them to be able to help me. Without him being there he wouldn't have known how to help me either? He helped a lot, because he could speak for me… When I couldn't? Since I didn't know what was happening to me? I couldn't always give them the answers that they needed. So, they could help me more either, and that's as important as the medications working properly, too! I often sometimes have a perverted sense of humor, too! I was told that most Epileptics do, too!

I don't know, but I do... Have that kind of humor, too! I've noticed it also, but I didn't notice it as much. Until my doctor told me what to look for before? Dr. Quinn told me what that was about? It's just a weirder sense of humor that's funny, but also can be perverted. That doesn't make me a bad person, but I'm corky! I'm not a sick individual like what you might think, because of that? I'm a sick person who struggles with health issues, and needs lots of things to help me. The VNS devices caused my voice to change a lot, and I couldn't sing without ending up with Laryngitis afterwards, too!

I still get Laryngitis when I sing? My voice gets harsher, but I'll have to use Cough Drops... To heal my scratchy throat, too! Since it bothers me, but I've always enjoyed singing! So, I don't let that stop me. Plus, I relax some doing it, too! Or it just helps me not feel so down or sad? Plus, it brightens up my day! I normally can pick up on the beat of the song, and it doesn't matter... If it's brand-new or not?

The beat, because I'm hard at hearing; and have trouble hearing music with my ears the way others do. So, it's by the rhythm, and I can pick up every song. I was involved in a lot of musical stuff... When I was a child, too? I played lots of instruments, and was in Band. I also played multiple instruments, but sang Professionally doing Gospel growing up, too! With my mama, and had a real good time doing that. I gave that up... When I left home, too? It was different, but only inside of Churches, Recording Studios & Radio Stations, too!

When I left home? I was on my own, and hadn't had anybody to look out for me? Except for God & myself, for a very long time, too! After I went into recovery? I had some more people that did care about me, and they looked out for me. Only when I'd let them? You can only do so much, but if a person won't let you help them? Then they have a harder walk to walk, and will make mistakes... Maybe taking them a lot longer to get to where they need, too? Before they reach their bottom? I reached mine, and that entirely changed my life, too!

I'm grateful for all of those people, too! Even if it was some that betrayed my trust, friendship & done me wrong? Why you might, ask? I still learned something from all of them, and I remained teachable, too! That helped me grow, too! I grew, blossomed and bloomed, into a young, beautiful woman… That was becoming aware of things she'd never known before about herself. Who had never been aware of the true meaning of love? Or about anything in life that had all been a delusion before! Why was it that way?

I was misguided, but in all the wrong directions… Except for a few, and that I'm really grateful for, too! I picked up learning from my grandparents & godparents, but also a few aunts & uncle's, too! That was important, because they were about doing… Right from wrong, and that's a big lesson to be learned. Especially being a child, and nobody teaching you anything, but bad things for the most part of your life. That gave me the strength that I needed, and talking to God… All the time helped me get through what I was going through, and coping with all alone? I managed being out on my own without any problems, but I still had plenty of problems, too! It was difficult for me, but I took chances playing with fire you could say?

Since I was taking chances being out going to places all alone? Due to not knowing… When I might go into convulsions or have seizures? Or something worse could happen to me, because of that? Being aware of the dangers, but not being willing to let anyone else… Be in control of my life, and being as independent. As what I could be on my own was very important to me? I didn't want to give up that responsibility for my freedom… Unless I didn't have a choice? I would I guess, I thought.

If that time ever comes, but not until then? Needless to say that time did come, and I wasn't very happy about it! It really upset me, too! Since I was used to going anywhere I wanted, too? Doing whatever I wanted, too? Without getting into trouble, and taking care of all the things I needed, too! Then I felt terrible, because I didn't have my independence… Having to depend on others to do things for me. That I used, too! It also affected my self-esteem, too!

Which wasn't very cool either, but I had to learn… How to deal with it all? That wasn't very easy either, but finally I got used to it some. Except it still bothers me even to this day, too! I used to enjoy going on those nature walks, riding buses, and going around the World… To places that I wanted, too! Now I can't necessarily do that, and it bites! Oh, well… That's life, and it's not always nice to you. Sometimes accepting what we don't want, too?

Can be overwhelming, but when we do? It's easier for us to manage & deal, with our problems. That's the hardest part sometimes, but it's worth it… Once you've gotten to that other side of it, and have moved past the problem right in front of you, too! Except sometimes it takes more time… To get a handle on some issues than others, but it's ok. Just never give up hope! That'll work, and help you through it… Plus, always remember that God's there, and he's never going to leave you! That he's always on your side, but have a support network, too!

That really helps a lot, too! Having a disorder that's a Neurological Disease called Epilepsy… Is very rough on everyone that's involved inside of your life around you. Sometimes it can be a major headache for your doctors, too! Since it can cause so many problems, but it's something that most of them know… Exactly how to handle? If they don't then you should find a new doctor that does know what to do? That's crucial to your health for one, and your life also. It's not an easy thing to manage at the beginning, but it can be that way… As long as it's an issue, too!

Having the right people to be there to help you is really important, and it helps make things more manageable, too! Since they'd know... What to do for you? What's best for you? Or what they might need to do next, too? When a person has Epilepsy it affects their whole body, but not just part of it. The brain is affected a lot, too! When seizures occur the brain misfires, and it can cause a person to not think the same way? Or it can cause them to not act the same way, too! It can also cause problems with focus, concentration & thought process being slower.

My Epilepsy & other seizures, that I've got that's been present my whole life... Have been a big struggle for me, but since I'm doing better on the medications for them. That I'm currently taking, and have to continue taking. I am able to do things that I wasn't able to do before... That I really wanted, too! Also, I'm still limited with some things, because of other issues... I still can't ever have a Driver's License, because my seizures can take place anytime. Plus, I'm not entirely seizure-free, but I'm aware... That I've been told that's probably never going to happen for me, too! That I'll never be completely seizure-free, because of the trauma that I endured as a child, too!

No matter how much medication I was to take that it wouldn't really matter much? My newest doctor has a different opinion about that, but he left it up to me... About increasing my medicine more, and I'm glad. Since I get to where I feel over medicated sometimes? Plus, I'm on so much medications already, and we didn't increase it anymore. Plus, it's caused me to gain weight that I didn't have before. There's always side-effects with these kinds of medications, and they're not always easy to deal with! I don't know, but I'm going with my best judgement; and that's what I decided? He was ok, too! With my decision of not increasing it anymore, and I'm glad.

That he wasn't going to force that, too! He's not a doctor that's like that, and he's very good at what he does, too? I'm really grateful that I've got him, too! He's helped continue the process that began before we moved here, and it's helping me… To move forward instead of going backwards! Which was what me, my spouse & his family, always wanted. Plus, a lot of other people in my life, too! I'm in a much better place than where I've ever been with my Epilepsy? Before in my entire life, but that doesn't mean… That I'm happy!

I struggle all the time sometimes, because of my problems; and them being difficult to handle. Plus, my Epilepsy & Seizures, have caused multiple other health problems for me, too! Which has made things even harder for me, but I'm still trudging along; and keeping up my faith & courage, too! That's something that can be hard often, too! Except you can do it, and I know that… If I can do it? Then anybody can do it! No matter how hard things get? Since I've managed to do it, but knew that it felt so impossible so many times; and I still made it through. It's easier said, than done that I also know.

I also believe that if you don't give up? You can make it to the point to where I've gotten, too? It's a journey that's hard, rocky, uneasy & miserable, too! It's also a remarkable amazing, strength, survivor & accomplishment… Along with being a success story or medical miracle, too! That's a miracle God gives to us, and helps us get past… The things that seem most impossible to do. I'm a medical miracle, but I used to be just a Science Experiment. At least that's how it felt? Since I was everyone's Guinea pig for so long.

I'm a miracle from God, too! If it wasn't for him? I wouldn't be alive today, and I am aware of that every day, too! I'm proud of myself, and the things… That I've been able to accomplish after getting my seizures under control? Plus, the things that I was able to accomplish before things worsened, but got so far out of control! Making it nearly impossible for me to function at all, and to live also… Making it difficult just getting up out of bed, and doing daily tasks. Since the seizures & Epilepsy, controlled my whole life. Plus, pretty much everything inside of it. Not allowing me to be able to be normal.

I felt anyways, because of my problems, and them making me feel… Like less of a person, too! So, many times, too! I'm successful at being able to accomplish some things… That's made me feel very good about myself. One was finishing school, but also getting a College Graduate Certificate, too! Then getting recognized as an Author, and being Published. Having a Certificate for that, too! Plus, my name being added onto a wall somewhere inside of Washington. Then being Published for the first-time last year through Amazon Self-Publishing & KDP.

You see I wasn't paid the first time I was published by a company that was called Madison's Who's Who? I was recognized as an Author & College Graduate, and granted a second Certificate of Recognition for myself; but also there was a Bibliography… That was short done about me in their book, too! It still made me feel very proud though, because it was a major accomplishment. Just like me being in recovery, too! Having 18 years of Recovery Time, and that's a big miracle, too! Everything happened for a reason, but I believe that God played the most important part… Of all the good things that's been happening inside of my life! I give him all the credit, and know that without him it wouldn't have been possible? Plus, my spouse has been very supportive to me, too!

That really means a lot to me also, because he's been there with me through all of this. That really was a great thing, too! Since he's been able to help me, but he put me through School also. I made him a promise… I was going to keep up doing what I wanted to do? I had to put it on hold for a while, but picked up my writing when I was able to return to it again? Even though it took me 9 ½ years, but at least I was finally able to pick it back up again! That's exactly what I'm doing, too! I'm doing what I'd originally set out to do, and feel really good about that also? That makes me really happy, too!

Especially since it's what I always wanted to be able to do? Plus, it's not as much about money, but yes… That does help, and I've not made a lot yet? I am glad that I've earned what I've been able, too? It makes me feel like I'm not wasting my time… Like some people will tell you often. It's still a work in progress, and I'm still a piece of work in progress, too!

Chapter 3. Side-Effects & Managing Them

So, everyone knows who has to take Epileptic Medications? That they've all got some serious side-effects, and that managing them... Can be a nightmare, too! That sometimes you've got multiple problems you've got to deal with... While trying to adjust to each one, but you can. Over time sometimes become able to manage them, and other times... They're too difficult to deal with, and the medications. Need to be changed, but that can also be something as simple as an adjustment. To your dose, too! One major problem is mood swings & suicidal thoughts, or feelings of suicide.

Deeper or worsening Depression, too! Then drowsiness, fatigue, restlessness, anxiety, hyperactivity or increase in seizures, too! Then sometimes there's the dry mouth which never usually goes away, but makes you always feel thirsty. Then there's the weight changes, but some medications cause weight loss; and some cause weight gain. It depends on what Regimen you have to take? Something that's not caused by the seizure medications, but the seizures themselves... Can be drooling, bladder loss, bowel incontinence, and nausea & vomiting, too! It can be really hard, but sometimes the medications can help with that also. Plus, your muscles can cramp up or get charlie horses in them, because of the seizures & medications, too! There can be loss of interest in things also, because of the seizures & medications, both.

Sometimes the side effects can be very overwhelming, and very uncomfortable… Trying to learn how to deal with them all? Especially when the medications & seizures, can cause you trouble dealing with multiple side effects & complications, too! It's not always comfortable trying to get through it either, and can be very difficult managing them all also. It takes time, but also giving yourself a break. When you're handling them, too? Since there's so many side effects that can be caused from dealing with the medications & seizures, too! They each have their own side effects of trying to cope with also… There's many ways in handling them, but sometimes you need support from others that understand what's going on with you also. So they can help you get through it, because you can't always easily get through it by yourself!

Then you've got your aftereffects, too! That's also very hard trying to handle… Or get a grip on, too? Since they can be very unmanageable trying to deal with also, and they can be overwhelming trying to handle. Since they can alter a lot of things inside of your life. Making things more complicated, but also more of a struggle… Than what you really wanted to have to deal with? Putting all kinds of obstacles in your way, and causing a whole bunch of extra problems, too! Making things even more difficult for you to control inside of your life. Coping with all these issues can be easy, but hard at the same time.

Since you've got to deal with so many issues, because of the side effects, aftereffects & seizures, too! Plus, you're trying to manage how they are causing things to happen inside your life, too! Sometimes you'll have really bad dry mouth symptoms to have to deal with, and loss of appetite. Plus, feeling dizzy or lightheaded, too! Then you'll have the grogginess, but feel hyper sometimes. You might have lots of mood swings to have to deal with, and that can be very frustrating. Plus, you might have severed light sensitivity, but also suffer with severe migraines, too! You sometimes might have an Aura, but other times… Maybe you won't at all, and have no idea when they're coming? A lot of times you'll have muscle aches, spasms & cramps, from them, too!

You can also throw up or feel like you're going, too! From the seizures & medications, too! Both of them can cause this to happen to you, but it's something that does pass. If it's related to these problems? Sometimes you can see spots, circles, or your vision will be very off… From what it normally is, because of side effects. Or from the seizures themselves? They can alter your eyesight a lot, too! That's just another part of it, but they can really interrupt your focus, train of thought, thought process, speech, and ability to concentrate. Your frame of mind state in general, because they can affect your brain so much.

Sometimes the way that it affects your mind will change, but return back to the way it normally functions somewhat; and maybe not all the way back to normal. What's normal for a person who has Epilepsy, and suffers from Seizures though? They can make you feel a lot of insecurity, too! They can cause you to have self-esteem issues, too! Which is often normal, but you can make it through that also. You can feel very depressed, because of them also, and need help with getting through that, too! You are generally a lot more emotional than what most people are, because Epileptics normally are like that. I've been told that's pretty normal though, and not to worry about it. Having Epilepsy can also cause other problems to happen to you, too! Which can make dealing with all the side effects even more difficult, and cause you to feel hopeless at times also.

It can be very frustrating, overwhelming, disturbing & uncomfortable, learning how to deal with this at first? When you're very first diagnosed? Not knowing what's going to happen to you, but also not being sure? About what to expect next? Later on it can feel the same exact way, too! Since there's usually more things that will come along, and often happen to you. Except not everyone will experience the exact same things, and may not feel exactly the same way. It's an individual based experience, but sometimes others don't go through... What someone else is? That's dealing with Epilepsy, because everyone's body is different; and everyone has a different experience.

Although they can experience and share, some of the same situations, problems, strength or hope, with others. Plus, their story can be similar, but maybe not everything they've gone through. Except you can still learn something from their experiences, and gain insight… On how to deal with your problems, too? That can be helpful in a lot of ways, because not everyone is so easy… To discuss these problems, because they're so different. From most problems & health issues, and can be very uncomfortable talking about, too! Sometimes people are ashamed, embarrassed or to upset, to even begin talking about them. That does take a whole lot of time, but you'll get there. If this is what's going on with you?

It's nothing to be ashamed or embarrassed, about either… Usually other people don't understand as much, but most people. Who suffer with Epilepsy can understand very quick? Plus, they can tell you… How cruel & mean, some people can be in life about things like this, too? Since they're usually just immature, because if they weren't? Then they'd understand that it's nothing to laugh about. Plus, it's not funny either! It's a very serious problem, and they are stupid… If they're making fun of someone, because they've got Epilepsy & Seizures, they're suffering from?

That's something that I've learned, but I had to learn that was the reason. That it's not your fault, because they don't understand something? That's happening to somebody, and that a person could die from it? Yes, that's true! It's no laughing matter at all, and it's actually a very serious disease… That can be fatal. No matter how long a person has being having seizures? Since there's a thing that's called SUDEP, too! It's when a person who has Epilepsy? Can die during a seizure, and pass on in their sleep, but sometimes somebody that's near you… Might be able to prevent you from dying.

If they catch this happening to you? They can call 911, and get you help when needed? I know that there's been multiple times that I've had to have help? Since I've almost died, because of my seizures. I've had those times, and my heart has completely stopped? Or I've turned blue, and had no pulse! When I've had to be revived, and resuscitated? Being brought back, because of my seizures almost taking me out of this World. No, having Epilepsy isn't fun at all, and it takes a lot of things away from you. That other people have no idea how hard that can be?

I've had so many near death experiences, because of my Seizures & Epilepsy, too! It's not even been pleasant at all dealing with! It's been very difficult, but I've managed to learn many ways of helping me cope. Sometimes that's easier than others, too! Since it can affect your mood so much, but make you stress out easily. Getting bent out of shape faster than the average person, and you put more pressure on yourself... Over trying to be more successful. At anything you're doing, too! Especially since others can make you feel like a failure a lot more easily, because you're an Epileptic. Blaming your or guilt tripping you, because of your problems.

Not to mention the fact, that it's easy enough... For an Epileptic to do this themselves, and they really don't need any help from others... Making them feel bad about themselves, because they can do that alone. Without anybody else's help! Being an Epileptic isn't easy for others around you... To deal with, and handle either! It can be overwhelming for them as the same with yourself, but they'll not give up on you. If they love you? Like your family, Spouse or Significant other... Is what I'm talking about.

It's a big commitment trying to deal with this with someone that has these problems, and it's something that's very worrisome to them also. They never know sometimes that you're going to be ok? Leaving them to deal with extra stress, too! Plus, they may not show you... How it's affecting them? Or they might be angry, because they don't like... What's happening to you? Just like you're angry sometimes, too! It's also a very big responsibility to handle, too! That often requires lots more attention than what you might want to give it, but is necessary for the person suffering with it.

It can be very tiresome on others, and not just the person that it's affecting, too! Epilepsy likes being in control of the person's life who has it? Sometimes that makes it harder for the person suffering with it, and those around them. Plus, their doctors, too! Since it can be so unmanageable, but after time? It can become a lot more manageable, and that's when greatness begins? Since it doesn't have the power or control, that it did before... Making it less powerful, but more manageable instead. That's when you can begin enjoying the little things inside your life? You've been missing out on until now?

When someone has Epilepsy? They've got a lot more to deal with on a daily basis... Than most people usually do, and no they're not the same kinds of lifestyles. Epilepsy can really limit an individual, and cause them to be homebound a lot... Depending on the situation, but then they can have sometimes where this might not be true? It depends on how you feel? How things are taking place in your life with it? Plus, how you're doing overall struggling more than others who have the same kind of health complication or not? Then other times you're allowed a little bit more freedom from the side effects, seizures, and aftereffects, too! That doesn't always mean that you're not going to have to depend on someone to be there for you or take you somewhere though?

I've been on so many different medications, because of my Epilepsy... I've had the disease since I was 13 years old, but that's only as far as I know? I was instructed that I could've had Epilepsy before then, but it wasn't diagnosed... Until I was 13 years old, because of whatever reasons? I was observed having seizure like activity before then... When I was a baby? I've slept through Tornados on several different occasions, because of my seizures... Making me sleep in such a deeper sleep, and being in a state of comatose state of mind sleeping. I've also slept through Straight line winds, and severe major thunderstorms, too! Nothing was going to wake me up until I was ready to wake up, because of my seizure activity?

I've been told that I wasn't ever going to get any better, too! That I was never going to be able to stop having as many seizures as what I was? Wrong!!! I'm doing so much better today, and my seizures are doing better today, too! I'm on a different combination of medications, but I'll probably never be completely seizure free. That's my dilemma, but I'm more manageable today... Since my seizures are better, and I'm doing better with my medications that I'm taking. Except for the fact, that I'm going to have some seizures; and they might not go away! My medication doesn't need to be increased anymore, because it's high enough on my dose as far as I'm concerned. What makes me so different?

I've got permanent scarring & bruising, on my skull & brain. From abuse being beaten in the head with hammers & car jack tools, because of my Adopted Dad. When I was a small child, and it lasted until I was 12 years old? I may never be completely seizure free, because of this... Is something that's being said, to me by previous doctors. Not my current doctor, but previous doctors, and I do also believe that. It's made things a lot more complicated, because of how they could treat me, too? Since it caused a lot of problems with doing certain things to help me... It's made it harder for me to be more aware of lots of things, because of the seizures, too! I'm a miracle that I even lived through what I did, and managed to survive it?

It's been a lot harder for me to accept the fact, that I will always have seizures... Due to this, too! I'm resentful, too! Only it's towards my Adopted Dad, because he damaged me for life. That'll never go away! Even though Epilepsy ran inside of my family, and on my Mom's side; but skipped every 3 generations. I was one of the generations that didn't get skipped, too! I also have more than just Epileptic Seizures, too! Which also makes it more difficult treating me, too! It's been a very tricky situation trying to find things to help me.

I've been everybody's guinea pig until recently? Reality is often harder to accept the truth, and deal with it... Than not wanting, too! Except if you don't deal with it? What else are you going to do? You can't ignore it, because it's not going to magically disappear. So, often I really wished that I could've made it magically disappear. I sure didn't want to accept the truth about it all one bit! It was extremely difficult to do, but once I did? It became a heck of a lot easier to understand everything.

I still find myself struggling often dealing with the side effects, aftereffects & how I feel? After my seizures, but also coping with the medications, too? That's no lie, and nope... That hasn't gotten very much easier at times to handle either! Also I've found that it's a thing that you've got to manage... When that happens, too? Not something that you can predict, because it won't affect you the same way every time either! Plus, it's one of those things that you've got to take... As it comes, and deal with it at the time being, too! Sometimes it's easier to deal with, but others it's harder to deal with; and that's just how it is I think?

I lean on God a lot, but that doesn't mean... That I don't lose my faith sometimes, and get lost. Being afraid, scared or frightened, about what's happening? When things can be so overwhelming, but yet difficult to get past? That doesn't mean that I don't bounce right back, but it sometimes can take more time... For me to do so, too! Often I feel like I'm on a rollercoaster ride, and am moving in all sorts of crazy directions; because of things. When I'm dealing with my Epilepsy? Plus, trying to manage & cope, with other things also... That may be causing me more problems to deal with, too!

Sometimes it's easier for me to handle, because I'm using music... To help me cope with my problems, too! It also can be very soothing, relaxing and uplifting, too! Plus, I enjoy having my animals or pets, around... They bring lots of joy into my life, and help me coping a lot also. They help a lot with dealing with my depression, too! Having support from others helps a lot, but I don't have as much of that... Now as what I used, too? Since the only person I really have that from is my Spouse, doctors & nurses, but they do understand. However they're not inside my body, and don't know what I feel like?

At least they do understand what I'm dealing with though? That's very important, and they might not be inside my body... Except they know from their medical teaching what I'm going through somewhat? That gives them a better idea, because they're educated about... What's going on with me? Which allows them to be able to help me more, too! Without their education & schooling, they'd not been able to do that. So, that's a very good thing that they are familiar with things that's going on, and can have an idea how to help? I'm very glad that they can, too! Since I'm the one who's dealing with these problems, but I also know that I'm not alone; because many people have these issues, too!

Sometimes you've just got to accept that you're going to have one of those days, and it may not be a good one. Since you've had seizures? Or because of your Epilepsy, but it'll get better. Sometimes it might just take more than a day for all of your symptoms... To go away, too! What's really bad? Is when you're having back to back sets of seizures, and they've been very bad? Making you feel pretty terrible, too! It also causes you a slower recovery time from dealing with the aftereffects, too. Since they've been so extreme & severe, but then they might not be so bad the next, time.

Or they could be? It just depends on how bad you're seizures are... When you're having them? I've been there, and I know... That's really hard to handle, too! It's not an easy thing to have to face, but it's very difficult. Making you feel really bad, and causing you multiple issues. Trying to deal with them all, too! It can be so exhausting, too! That's one thing they'll do to you quick, but you can get past that also.

It doesn't happen overnight either, and can be very hard moving forward with, too! Prayer, meditation, faith, courage & support, are all very important. When dealing with issues like this? Plus, having a support network can be very useful, too! Since it can be an outlet for you, and others… That are trying to deal with these problems that you're having in your life. Sometimes you can have little, but a little is all that you need. As long as you've got some… I believe that you'll be ok. Fear, anxiety, worry, overwhelming insecurities, can override how you're really feeling sometimes also.

Don't let it all get to you, and take over; because what you're going through will pass? I just can't tell you when? It's easy to do, and let it all get to you also; because I know how easy it is to stress when you're an Epileptic? Epileptics have more tendency to stress a lot easier… Than what the average person does? Plus, they've a harder time dealing with things in general, and it isn't always a smooth ride. Handling problems that arise inside your life, but trying to maintain a positive attitude… About everything, too! It's easier to get more depressed, too! Accomplishments often mean more to you though, because everyone can be so hard on you; and make you feel less than.

So, can yourself be hard on yourself… As much as other people can be, too! That's just part of how it is? It doesn't really matter who it is? Since you're sometimes the person who knows you the best? That can beat up on themselves better than anyone else, too! It's so easy for you to do, because you can't see… What you're doing sometimes? Except you know, and realize it at some point. That's when you stop it?

So, when you stop beating yourself up? What's your next, move? You look for all the things that you can be grateful for, and you make a note of them all. Then you start doing something that will help make you feel better? Plus, you have to retrain your brain, and help it change... Those negative thoughts into some positive thoughts, and that's not always easy to do either. Except if you're patient enough? You don't give up, and keep working on it... Then you can do it! If I can do it then you can, too?

Even when I'm struggling, but fighting with myself... I can do it! So, can you, because you can learn how to? It's like being programmed or being a program, but changing that... What it does, and how it works? So, that you're different without doing things that can make you feel worse about yourself. You just simply start out slowly, and work on one thing... To change at a time, but after time. You'll be able to make a lot of changes, and that'll definitely make you feel a whole lot better about yourself, too! It gives you a brand-new outlook on your life, too!

After you've been able to start doing this? It'll help you with your self-esteem, too! Plus, it's something that will help your attitude, but there's still times... That might be an issue that you'll have to deal with, because of the seizures & side effects, of the medications, too! It does get better, but it doesn't seem like it sometimes. Since that's something that it feels like you've always got to work on, because of what's happening to you? It does affect your attitude a lot, and there's no way around that I don't think. It gets easier though to deal with, but it still is something that is progress. It doesn't happen overnight either! How much time it takes depends on how bad it is also?

For everyone that's something that is also very different, and it may not be the same... For some individuals that it is for others, but everyone's attitude is affected. Whether or not? They really want to tell the truth and admit, that? That's just how it is? Why? I'm not really sure, but it's also nerve-wracking to have to worry about, too! Everyone has pretty much got to accept that you're not to be not treated unequal, because of your problems. They should still treat you equally, because you're just as important as anyone else also. Plus, you're not really any different from anyone else; because you're a person like everyone else is, too!

It's just that, because you're an Epileptic & seizures, you're some different. That doesn't mean that you should be treated different, because you're an Epileptic; but in some cases that does. It depends on what the circumstances are? What I mean is this? It's a problem, but you shouldn't be treated unequal over it... Sometimes there's things that are handled a lot differently, because of you being an Epileptic & having seizures. That's what I was trying to say? Things are a lot more sensitive, and so are you sometimes... When it comes to dealing with things, too? So, that means that your needs are handled with a lot more care most of the time, because of that also.

That's ok though, because your needs are a lot different than most peoples, too! Which makes things sometimes more difficult, but also take a lot more time. That's also something that's ok, and there's nothing wrong with it. You're not a defect! You're not a mistake!!! Plus, you're not stupid or weak! All due to the fact, that you've got Epilepsy. Just because some people don't understand what that's like? That's their problem, and not yours! That just means that they aren't familiar enough to know what's wrong with you, and they should learn what it's about?

Chapter 4. My Journey

My journey with my Epilepsy hasn't been very pleasant, but I know… That I'm not any different than anyone else who suffers with this sort of illness, and I'm not unique due to having been diagnosed with Epilepsy. Except I often struggle a lot more with things than a lot of people. Most people who do have Epilepsy usually do… From what I've been told by doctors before, too? It's pretty normal, and it's very overwhelming at times; because I'm more emotional than what I'd like to be? I'm moodier with my seizures, but for the most part now… It's not as bad as what that used to be! Especially since my seizures are much better controlled now, and I'm doing a lot better with them. Than what I've ever done my whole entire life?

That doesn't mean that there's still not days where I'm having difficulty? Where I'm feeling totally crappy, but am doing my best to hang in there? Even when it seems like it's, too difficult? I know that I'm always going to have my good days, but also my bad days, too! When the seizures happen, and it also depends on how bad of an effect they have on me afterwards? That varies, but often it does… That's just the way that it works with having Epilepsy. Nobody can really predict the outcome of that, but you know how you feel generally before & after? That's always important, too! Since you're not going to feel the exact same way that you did before, because the seizures make you feel pretty awful!

That's a part of having Epilepsy that can make things become more uncontrollable. The part that doesn't always seem to help you, but sometimes can make a difference... In your life, because you can journal. How you're feeling before & after, and learn from that also? About what's happening to you with your seizure activity. To help explain things more for yourself, but also your doctors, too! It actually isn't a bad idea either... From what I've learned? I've had to do it with others helping me the best they could keeping track of my seizure activity, and that wasn't very easy to do. Sometimes nights, days, evenings or afternoons can blend, together.

Making that nearly impossible to do. Since the seizures can often be so bad... That it can cause lack of sleep for anyone that's around, and lots of confusion, too! That's another part of it also, but when the seizures are under better control? It doesn't make that much of an impact on everyone, but the person having them. Most of the time, unless you're seizing so bad... You're waking up somebody? Then it can affect the sleep the same way, and there's not a lot that can be done about that sometimes. Seizures happen whenever they're going to happen? That's another thing that's unpredictable with them, too!

There's been a lot of things inside my life... That I wanted to do, but couldn't enjoy. Due to me being an Epileptic, and I'd still sometimes do them anyway; but I'd pay a price for that. Like going to Concerts, Firework Shows, and things like that... They'd cause my seizures to be worse, because of all the flashing lights; and I'd have a really hard time afterwards. Having multiple sets of seizures & back to back episodes, until they decided to quit? Whenever that would be? I'd feel so terrible afterwards, and couldn't function at all! I wouldn't even be able to cook sometimes, do housework, or daily chores & activities, that I needed to finish. The price I'd pay for a little bit of fun & entertainment, wasn't really good; because of my Epilepsy.

Even though it was at the time when I was trying to enjoy myself at a Concert & Fireworks Show? It just caused me to have some really bad problems afterwards, and I had to deal with them. That's all, but it wasn't just myself; because my Spouse also had to deal with them, too! Since he was the one who had gone with me, but knew that I might have seizures... Knowing that it may not happen right away, but that it could happen fast, too! That's something we never knew, and still don't. Since I've got multiple types of seizures, and they all appear to look similar; but aren't... It makes it harder to tell what kind I'm having when I'm having them? Unless you've done a test on me that's a Video EEG, and they've done those; but learned there's more than one kind. I have 4 types of seizure disorders: Grandma Epileptic, Partial Onset Epileptic, Non-Epileptic Partial & Pseudo Seizures, too!

So, I'm an Epileptic with Non-Epileptic Seizures, too! Which makes it a lot harder to treat me, but my doctor isn't having any trouble doing that. Which is very good, but it took forever in my life... To find doctors that were able to start helping me, and that didn't happen until about 5 ½ years ago? Then my current Neurologist was able to finish what the other doctor started? Which has been very good for me, too! It's helped me in so many ways, because I was in really bad shape. Just from my Epilepsy by itself, and it's caused me multiple other health issues, too! Which is really bad, but I'm trying to take care of everything the best that I can; and with my doctors help also. Since there's multiple issues to deal with, but also not give up.

Sometimes I really feel like doing that, because it's so depressing, hard, and aggravating except I don't! I've fought my whole life to stay alive, because I didn't want to let anything win or anyone win. From what's happened to me, and what I've been through? So, I wasn't going to give up no matter how much I wanted, too? I was going to come out the winner on the other side I always told myself... No matter how much it hurt! I wasn't going to let anybody else have that power, and take away my life! They weren't going to get what they wanted, too? For a really long-time having Epilepsy felt like I had a Curse! That I was completely doomed, and beyond help at all.

Why? Others including many doctors made me feel this way, because they really didn't know... What to do to help me? Or they had the attitude that they didn't care, and wasn't going to even attempt to try to help me? That there wasn't anything they could do for me, and that there wasn't any hope for me. Or that they'd given up entirely on helping me get better at all? They were done! They weren't going to try anymore, and that was very hard for me to accept. I wasn't going to accept it either, because I wasn't ready to give up on myself! I was going to do whatever it took to get better?

Sometimes that wasn't as easy said, or thought... As what I'd hoped for? I didn't give up though, and kept trying until? I was able to find the right doctors to help me? That took a whole lot of time, but I finally accomplished doing that also. Then things in my life slowly started turning around. For a while it was very slow, but then finally... Things sped up, and it was all turning around so fast. I could hardly believe it! It was like a dream come true, because everyone had said, that it wouldn't happen before!

When it did? I was shocked, too! I almost didn't believe it, because it didn't seem real at first... It almost seemed, too good to be true! Except it wasn't so, because it was really true! That was a great feeling inside, too! Especially after knowing what I've gone through my entire whole life? It hadn't been easy at all, but lots of people had given me a very hard time over it. Misdiagnosing me, being mean, and not being there to help me! Plus, even some people making lots of fun of me, because I was an Epileptic.

It's not funny! It really made me feel so good knowing that things were starting to look up for me. Knowing that my life was going to change, but was it going to be enough? To make everything better inside my life? No, was the answer on that one... That didn't mean that I needed to give up though, because that just meant there was still going to be lots of problems to deal with & handle. I was going to need a lot more attention & medical requirements, because of all my problems. Getting the seizures in under better control... Wasn't going to make a big enough difference in my life the way everyone had hoped that it would? I was still going to have lots of battles, obstacles & things to cause me lots of difficulty... Keeping me from getting a lot of things in order the way I even wanted, too!

That really made me angry, disgruntled & unhappy, too! There was enough extra problems that was caused, because of my Epilepsy; and that didn't help either! Making it even harder for all of my problems to get better. That doesn't mean that they won't ever improve, but lets face it... I'm 45 years old now, and by the time they do. If they ever did? It might be, too late! I might not have that much life left inside of me, because I've got some serious problems... That could make that very possibly true. That doesn't mean that I'm right either, but I feel that my time isn't long left here on this place called Earth; and I feel that way due to many problems I'm not going to mention here.

I was just telling my Spouse... That I feel tired, and I'm ready to go. When God lets me go, because I'm tired... I don't know how much more fight I've got left inside of my body? I really don't, because things have taken a toll on me; and I'm exhausted. I'm weaker than what I should be? Due to my problems, and I don't get around... As good as what I'd like, because of how everything has affected me & my body through the years? It's really made me very fragile, and I'm not in good health... With multiple health issues to deal with daily, but at the same time doing my best to hang in there.

Even though it feels almost impossible sometimes, too! When I talked to him about how I felt? I also let him know... That I love him very much, and that I never wanted him to forget that! Since I don't always feel like I might be here from one day to the next, but wanted to make sure... That he knew that no matter how hard things have been on both of us? We've always had a really hard time, because of a lot of my medical issues. It's not been real easy to deal with, and it's put us in Financial Debt also... Especially when we didn't have Insurance to always help? Medical Bills can pile up very easy, and our Government doesn't care about people who are sick!

Since all they mostly care about is themselves, and not taking care of people who need it? Or helping those that are hurting, but need help the most! Sometimes you're damned if you do, and damned if you don't? Well that's so true! Or you've got to pick and choose, what you're going to go with or without? In order to have what you need? Or you're neglected, because you can't get the help you need... Due to lack of money, doctors & Insurance. That doesn't make things right either! Sometimes it just doesn't work out for you, because of all of this; and if you do get help?

You're judged or looked down upon or not taken care of properly, too! Being that you can get a hold of some really bad doctors anywhere? That doesn't really matter, because sometimes it's just that people don't really care. That's what I've come across, and no it isn't right... Except it does happen! Whether or not people want to admit it or not? It's so very true, because it happens more than it's often talked about. Why? People don't like telling the truth all the time, and that's why it's not mentioned that much? I'm sorry, I don't believe in sugarcoating anything for nobody; because I believe in what's true?

I don't believe that a person should have to worry about getting the help they need. Or what they're going to do about getting food, medication, or personal hygiene items? Or which bills they can afford to pay, because of medical needs, and medications that they need. It just isn't right! Or if they're going to have to do without a whole bunch of things, because their medicine is so high... They can't afford anything else hardly at all? That's just not cool, but that's the place that lots of people are in; and these Pharmaceutical Companies should be made to lower prices on all these medications. Since it's peoples lives that are at stake, because of it all! They're the ones ripping people off, and these Insurance Companies are just as bad; because they just take advantage of people. With unaffordable Deductibles & Charges, they won't take care of... That they are supposed, too!

They're both like Con-Artists in ways, because they take so much advantage of you... By how much money they take away from you & your family! Not really caring about you, and your family being able to survive... Or have what you need? Honestly the Pharmaceutical Companies & Insurance Companies, don't care if you live or die? That's the whole truth about the matter, because they're selfish... In all of it for the money, and that's it! So, you need to have some people on your side who do? Or you're in some big trouble, because without that support... You can't stand alone, and it's not good for you!

That's just a cold hard fact about the sad truth on how everything is... Due to the fact that the Pharmaceutical Companies & Insurance Companies, are only in everything they do for the money. I really didn't mean for this to turn out seeming like a bitch session either, but I did need to vent my feelings. Since it's something that's really affected me & my husband, because of my health issues. I know first-hand about how they do treat you over needing your medications? Plus, how they make it almost financially impossible to get them sometimes, too! Both are to blame for how they take advantage of household families, and people that must take medications... Or get health care, because they've got to have it! It's a necessity, and something that everyone needs also. I wasn't sure exactly what all was going to come out in this Book, but I'm glad that I can express how I feel, too?

Sometimes things can come out when you're doing a True, Life, Meaningful Book… That you might not expect, but that's ok. The truth is better than a lie! I do believe that, but it doesn't always feel like that; because sometimes others can make you feel bad… For telling the truth, but I'd rather be truthful instead of dishonest about anything. That's just how I am? I don't like being dishonest, and I don't keep secrets for anyone… Unless it's a matter of life & death, because they're in danger? Sometimes there's those situations, too! That can be hard on somebody who has Epilepsy?

Since they've got some tough decisions to make on what's the best thing to do? I don't struggle with that one though, because life's taught me how to handle it? I must say that being abused as a child, and being severely beaten… Didn't help me recover with any of my Epilepsy Seizures that's not part of the ones they can control. It really hurt me more than anything, but I'm the one who's had to live with that my entire life? I'm the one that's had to be everyone's Guinea pig, and go through all this crap… I really wished that I never had to ever had gone through, but I didn't have a choice! Plus, I know that I'm not alone, because other people suffer with having the disease of Epilepsy; and it's not a pleasant journey to have to go down either. That does help make you not feel so bad, because you know others have it; and have been dealing with it just like you. Or they might be a friend or somebody, that's an outlet that you can talk to also?

What the beatings did do? Was leave me with a severe brain injury, and damage that's nonreversible. I'm managing though, but I'm also doing a lot better... Than what everyone ever said, I would do, too? Since my doctor has been able to get my seizures under better control, and get me on the right combination of Anti-Epileptic Drugs... That I've got to take, but with them I'm better stabilized; and I can do the things I wanted to do before they were so far out of control. Except I've days where I struggle doing a lot of things, too? Sometimes it's not always from my seizures, but I'm not having them all the time... Now the way that I used, too! Just since I'm an Epileptic it doesn't make me crazy either, but I'm moodier than most people.

Most Epileptics are moodier than most people, but sometimes the medications... That you take for your seizures are very helpful with that, too! As long as you're not put on anything that doesn't agree with you. If that's the case? Then there might need to be some more changes to be made. So, you're feeling better, and doing much better than... What you are? Instability with any Epileptic is a very bad thing, too! So, is unmanageability also, because it doesn't help you heal the way you need. Plus, it can cause major setbacks, too!

It also will benefit you a lot more... If you're taking the proper medications? To treat your seizures when they're Epileptic Seizures? Plus, there's medications they use to treat the other ones also, and it often... Takes more than one medicine in most cases, because of them being so bad. Or happening so frequently? Causing so many issues for the person who has the Seizure Disorders & Epilepsy? It helps when you've a doctor who can help? That is very familiar with everything about the disease, and how to treat your problems, too? That's very important, because I've not always had that; and that did more harm than good for my health & Epilepsy.

Trust me on that, because I know from my own experiences! How important that is, and why you should? Have the proper care, but you're not always going to be able to find it? Where you think you might? That makes it a lot more difficult, too! The cost & care, can be a very big deal for you & family, too! It's not something that's very affordable, and can cause a lot of hardship on everyone inside your household. It's not a burden, but it's a problem that needs a lot of patience, understanding, comfort for the patient & support. That does make things a lot easier, too! Having faith, trust & believing in God... Helps out a lot also, but that's everyone's own choice.

I know that it's helped me a lot, because without his help? I wouldn't probably be here, and I'm aware of that fact. I often wonder sometimes... Why? He's spared me so many times, because I've had so many near death experiences. I'm not saying that to frighten anyone, but it's true. I know today why? He's got a purpose for me in life, and it's not time for me to go home to be with him. That I'm still a piece of work in progress, but I've got more life inside of me; and he's not ready to take me yet? That's his decision, but when that time comes?

I'm at peace with it all, because I know that's it going to be ok; and I know where I'll be? That's going to be right there up inside of Heaven with him, and family, and pets I've lost... Along with my Spouse, because I'm sure I'll go before he does. Why would I say that? I know, because of my health; and how I'm with all the problems I have to deal with all the time. With my health issues, but also by God telling me so! That's something I've got his word on. When I died, and was standing outside my bod? During one of my VNS Implants, I was in Heaven. He told me then that he wasn't ready for me, because he had a purpose for me to finish.

I've figured out what that purpose is? Only my health isn't the best, and I know that in time my time will come to the final end; but I'll be at peace. During my first VNS Implant surgery I almost didn't make it out, but he brought me back. Along with the surgical team & doctors and nurses, too! I was in surgery for over 6 hours, but then later released to go home. My second surgery went a lot smoother, but my VNS Implant failed me, and when it did? I almost died again, because I went into Epileptic Seizures; and I wasn't coming out? I wasn't aware of anything that was going on around me, and I didn't know what'd happened to me? I didn't know how I'd even gotten to the hospital? It sure wasn't funny!

That's why I'm so glad & relieved, that my new doctor won't make me go through... Having another implant put inside of me. We found out that my VNS Implant is broken, too! It must've gotten broken when I'd had seizures? After it was shutoff due to failing & malfunction, but there's a lot more danger of them... Completely removing it than leaving it inside of me like that, because it's been shutoff. It can't do anything especially now being broken & off. It's just a pain, and causes discomforting chest pains. It still moves around a lot, too! If they were to remove it?

I could die? I don't want to die, and they'd not be able to remove everything; because they'd still have to leave a piece of the wire inside that goes to my brain. This is the really sad part... The second VNS Implant did actually seem like it was starting to help me some. Except they weren't able to turn it up all the way like the first one, because of all the pain it caused. Until it malfunctioned & failed, when I needed it the most? The first one just always malfunctioned, and caused me some permanent damage that's irreversible, too! So, I've got to also deal with that as well. Now though with the two seizure combination medications I'm taking... I don't need the devices anymore!

I'm so glad to know that now, too! If I had it to do all over again? I wouldn't have had the devices put inside my body at all, because of what I know now! Knowing that I wasn't given much choice at the time, because I was told... I wouldn't be eligible for the device in the future. If I didn't have the surgery? I prayed about it for 6 months before making a decision? I really wasn't sure what to do, but pray over it all? It's a really big deal! The biggest complication is death & resuscitation, during the very first surgery.

Or risk of a Heart Attack & Stroke? Those are some pretty serious things to really think about, but you've also got to worry about a possible blood transfusion if needed? You can bleed to death during the surgical procedure, because of how you've got to be cut open for the placement of the devices! Everyone has a decision sometimes that's difficult to make, but the VNS Implant I wish I'd never made. Especially with all the extra problems it's caused me to have, and they're not fixable! I also was told I'd lose my Insurance, too! If I didn't have the surgery? When I had my first surgery? I had glue put on my neck & throat, but also over my chest... Where the cuts were made for the device placement?

To keep me from bleeding to death! They do this to all the patients who have the surgery for it, too! I had staples & stitches, both... Dried blood all over my neck & throat, but also my chest. I wasn't allowed to shower or bathe... For 3 days after surgery, and had to be watched. By my spouse, and he had to feed me... Help me get dressed & showered, too! When I could go get cleaned up? I couldn't move my arm & shoulder, but also had to be very careful... Not to pull anything loose where I had staples & stitches.

It really makes you feel gross, because of having to wait. Except there's a reason, and that's the risk of surgical infection if you don't listen? So, you're better off to listen & follow, doctors orders upon release from the hospital. Since it's so important that you do, because you certainly don't want? To get an infection that's a Staff Infection from surgery. I hear that's a terrible thing, but it's also something… I've never had, because I follow doctors' orders! I'm a very slow healer, and it took me a lot longer to heal up. Plus, they had to pop my shoulder & arm, back in place, too! It got stiff with me laying on top of the operating table the way I had to do?

There's no way around that, but it does really stink; because it's painful. I also don't have a very high pain tolerance level, and have been through a lot… That has made that more difficult for me to handle, too! Sometimes that just happens that way, but everyone is different. Nobody can tell me that you're not going to feel pain… After going through that? You certainly are, and no it's not something very comfortable at all! It hurts very bad, too! It does get better, but then you've got to adjust to having pain from the device also. Plus, when they turn them on? That causes pain, too!

Chapter 5. How I Feel

I have a lot of feelings about this, and how I actually do feel? For one I'm not very healthy, but also have other problems… Due to my Epilepsy, and the seizures being so far out of control before. For so long, because they weren't successfully taken care of by the medications that'd been used. Plus, due to me not always having the right doctor's to take care of me also. Sometimes it was the fact the kind of Insurance I had, or if I had any at all? That also played a very big part in my care, too! Plus, I've got a bunch of other health issues to deal with also that doesn't have anything to do with my Epilepsy. Except it makes things harder for me to deal with, and things inside my life a whole lot more complicated, too! It also makes things a lot less likely for me to ever achieve a lot of things I really wanted, too!

I do keep trying to do some things I really wanted to do though, but there's some things… That I've had to completely not continue, because of health complications. It was for my best interest & benefit, because I have to take care of myself… The very best that I can, and that sometimes does mean. You might not be able to do some things you want to do? As far as Sports & things, like that. Since there may be other things why you've been told not to do them… From your doctor's & physician's, because they're only trying to look out for you also. To prevent any further issues that you could have complications from? That doesn't mean that you have to always like being told that, but you accept it; and find something else you can do.

Since that doesn't mean that you have to give up everything, but certain things sometimes. Like I had to stop going Bowling, because I became unable to do it anymore. I was also told by my doctor's & physician's, that it was best… If I didn't continue doing it anymore? Why? Due to some heart problems, nerve damage problems, and a few other problems, too! At first I was told by a Neurologist that it'd be very good for me, but if I started having problems? I should stop immediately! I struggled a lot, but I still tried. Until I was made to stop?

You see, I've got Peripheral Neuropathy & Fibromyalgia, too! Which can be very painful, but doing sport activities can also help… Unless it becomes very unmanageable? Mine did, and I developed heart problems; because of my Epilepsy & Seizures. That I was having so much, because they were so far out of control; and unmanageable for so long, too! That's what happened, but I also had 2 strokes; because of my seizures? They happened after my seizures, and I didn't receive medical attention right away; because I didn't have any medical insurance. That's what happened? That's the truth, but there wasn't anything that I could do about it. I had also been trying to work a job, because everyone said, that's what I needed to be doing?

I knew what the outcome was going to be? Except I was bound and determined, to do it anyway! Just to prove to everybody that I wasn't a loser or a bum… I got tired of hearing them all say that, and it was very painful! It made me angry, resentful, but very bitterly upset with them. I withdrew inside, and I wouldn't talk to anyone about how I felt? I just took it out on myself, and others around me. With angry outbursts that I had to learn how to control? Finally, I did over time… I stopped doing that for the most part, but I still stood up for myself.

I wasn't going to let anyone run over me, and be so mean to me! The way that they were before, but I wasn't able to work. Everyone knew that, but I tried it anyway. I still finished schooling, and got my Diploma. Being a Graduate made me feel pretty good, too! Even if it was taking schooling at home, and getting my Diploma. That was a really big deal, but I'm also very glad that I was able to do it, too! I had a lot of people that were very proud of me, too! I really was also, but I was very happy that my Spouse... Was very proud of me, too!

He knew how hard I tried & worked, getting through my schooling? So, did my College Instructor, and she was very proud of me also. A lot of my friends were really proud of me, too! That really did make me feel good inside, but I wasn't finished yet? I was just getting started, but then suddenly... Something terrible happened to me, and I had seizures very bad? I suffered a stroke, and I didn't successfully complete what I'd planned on doing? I was able to finally pick up where I left off, and start fresh 9 ½ years later. Putting my Author Career on hold, and having to set it to the side; because of my Epilepsy & Strokes, that occurred afterwards. I really didn't want to take a break that long, but I'm glad I've been able to get back to it all now!

That really makes me feel very happy! Especially since I've a natural gift. That's what I was told by my College Instructor, too? She said, that I had a natural gift & talent; because she'd seen it in some of her Students before. Not everyone does have a natural talent & gift, for something... That's something to be very proud of, too! People may laugh at me, but I don't care! I know that I'm very talented. I really don't care... What they think about me, because I believe in myself, too?

I know I'm capable of sitting down, and writing a Book about anything. I've been doing that, and I only started by doing Children & Teenager's Stories, Articles & Books. During that process, I learned how to write for Adults, too! When I picked back up? I started with all Adult stuff, and then broke everything down mixing it all up a bit. The aftereffects of my seizures sometimes... Changes my whole outlook on things, because it can cause me to feel like a failure. When I know, that I'm not? That's just a part of it that I've had to learn how to deal with? It's a thing you're going to have to learn how to cope with on your own, because everyone is different that has Epilepsy.

It's something that seizures can often & will, do a lot in people who have the disease of Epilepsy, too? Everyone has a different way of coping, and I've got many different ways I cope. Sometimes it's not always easy, but it's better when the time passes? That you don't feel so glum after your episodes, because they can take all the good out of everything sometimes, too! That's another part of Epilepsy that I don't like, but it's true. Often more than not enough times it's just difficult getting through the day, and the nights also... When you're seizing? It causes me to feel pretty bad still so now, but my seizures are also better controlled. That didn't make everything go away, because they are though. It just let me be able to do things inside my life somewhat differently than before, and made some things easier; but not everything for me is easier.

Since it still does cause problems in my life, but I can manage things a lot better than before. Most of the time, but it also depends on how bad the seizures are, too? If they're not light & mild, then they can still make me feel the same way as before. That's just how they operate? It's something that I'm still totally unaware of. When they happen? Or when I've had them, but I'm usually feeling pretty bad afterwards? Sometimes I can tell by that, but sometimes others will let me know. That I've had some seizures, and I might be feeling bad due to that happening. I have to take things as they come, and not get, too far ahead of myself.

Since I don't know when they're coming most of the time also? I don't always have a warning sign before they happen called an aura. It depends on what I can do sometimes, because of the way I'm feeling? After I've had my seizures, too! Plus, the rest of the time I'm limited on what I can do also? Having limitations doesn't mean that I'm totally helpless, but that I can't do things that maybe others can. It makes me feel bad, and I get down about it a lot of times also. Plus, I have to find ways of dealing with that, because it can depress me really bad. I get frustrated of having to take my medications, but I know… I don't have a choice, because if I didn't?

I could possibly go into seizures and die, because they've been that way so many times; and out of control almost causing me to do exactly that, too! I'm proud of the things that I've been able to accomplish in my life also, because it means a lot to me. Especially knowing what I've been through, and how much I've had to deal with these problems getting in my way, too? I know that taking care of yourself, and also following doctor's orders… Is very important when it comes to trying to get a handle on Epilepsy? Except that's with any kind of disease, because if you don't? You're going to have trouble not getting any better at all, but that's not what I wanted? I wanted to get better, but I'm not 100 percent better, because I've still got plenty of problems to handle on a daily basis. I try not to get, too overwhelmed dealing with it all. Sometimes that happens, and I need a little bit of extra encouragement & TLC.

Sometimes I have to do something nice for myself… In order for me to feel better, too! It actually does work though, and I can feel better then. Even if it's just taking a break, because I need to regroup… How I'm feeling, and get my mind-frame back to normal again? That can make a whole lot of difference, but then there's other things… Sometimes that I have to do, too! That's just finding ways to relax. Oh, that's a big one for me… Since I have a hard time of relaxing, but sometimes I can manage to relax a little bit.

A little bit is better than none at all though. I usually can always mostly relax with music anytime, but not if I've had some of my seizures. I don't feel nearly as good, and usually am not in the mood as much for it! That's just how I feel with mine sometimes, but it's not just music that I feel that way about. It can be about everything, and I don't want to be bothered by anybody either. Since they make me feel like I should shy away from others, and stay to myself more. Isolating myself, but yet being in my own comfort zone. Right where I love to be? It makes me feel safer that way, too! I've always had some walls around me, because I built them a long time ago to keep others out in a way of protecting myself.

There's other reasons for that, too! It doesn't really matter, but the main thing… Is that I feel safe & protected, that way. That's what matters to me, but I also realize? That's not always what is best for me, because I'm isolating myself? Which is true, and everyone needs people in their lives, too! It's easy to keep people out though, and not let many people in… Especially when you feel like they might look down on you? Due to you being an Epileptic, but maybe they're not so judgmental. Maybe they won't treat you mean, because they don't hold that against you in any way?

Maybe they'll be a better friend or acquaintance, to have inside your life? Plus, they might have some things they share with you, and it can help make you feel better? Sometimes that's the case, but it doesn't always work out that way. Usually when others share things with you, because they can let you know something about them… That's not something they let everyone know it can help you by being able to open up a little bit. You don't have to open up to others right away all at once, and sometimes… It doesn't really matter if you do or not? It won't change anything in some circumstances, but that's ok, too! I know from my own experiences that it's a lot easier to do things slowly, because you've got to be careful… Who you trust also?

That pretty much goes with everything and everybody, too! Inside of life, because some people can't be trusted at all… That goes without saying, and sometimes we learn the hard way over that one, too! It doesn't make it less easy if someone breaks your trust, and hurts you? After you've started trying to open up, and express things about yourself… Sharing about things in your life that aren't easy to cope with. I've learned that when this happens? Don't trust that person anymore with anything ever again, because they really weren't someone… You needed inside your life to begin with. If they act like that?

That's not an easy lesson to learn in life, but it's definitely a good one… Especially since there's people who just want to be mean to others, and don't have any respect at all for anyone else. Of course, it's better knowing who you can trust? Instead of learning the hard way, but that happens. If it does? Don't sweat it, because you've got to move forward… Don't let them win, and have control or power; over how you feel about yourself? They aren't worth it, but you're worth every bit of effort that you put into yourself & life; because you're the most important person around. That counts on being there for everything to work out for the best inside your life the most! Always remember even if that sounds cocky that you're an important person, and you shouldn't give up on yourself since you matter so much?

You need to be strong for yourself, and everyone around you that matters the most to you also. If you're not? Then you can't be there for yourself & them, too! Plus, you want to get better & improve… Don't you want that the most? Then do what you've got to in order to help that process begin? Or you might not get any better if you don't? I believe that most everyone wants to get better, but I also know that fear, anxiety & panic, can set in. Making you feel hopeless, too! Don't give up, because there's hope for everyone no matter how bad things are?

At least that's what I believe, because that's happened for me? When I was told that it wouldn't ever happen inside my life at all? That I had doctors give up on me, and told me there wasn't anything else that they could do for me. Except there was, but they didn't want, too! Or just flat out didn't care, too! I don't believe that there's not hope for nobody, because everyone should have that to hold onto. That's an important part of your recovery & healing process, too! It makes a World of difference, because that gives you some peace of mind; and it helps your attitude to have a better opinion about how you're going to do? Which is a good thing, because it's your life… Epilepsy has been controlling it, and taking over; but not anymore!

All that did when it happened? Had really upset me, and make me feel very angry. Especially when I found out that there was something that could be done to help me, and that some people just hadn't cared as much to help me? The way that I needed to be helped, because of my problems with Epilepsy being so severe. Then I felt this amazing, warm feeling coming over me; because I had some hope again. It wasn't over, but just getting started; and there was a lot more work to be done. Before I was going to be getting any better? I didn't always understand what was being said, to me either… About the problems & conditions, that I was dealing with; but I was willing to learn. I had one doctor say that it takes a lot of patience dealing with a person who's an Epileptic, and he's exactly right it certainly does!

He also told me that it takes a lot of understanding, work, time & effort, to do… What needs to be done in a lot of cases, too? Since it's not an easy thing to always treat, and can be very frustrating. He's right about that, too! Plus, it can be very time consuming, because there's so many things to deal with; and try to tackle all at once also. Sometimes it's not as simple as a medication adjustment, and takes longer to fix these issues. It's also very inpatient dealing with these problems, because the person who has them? Doesn't always feel like their best interest is at stake, and is confused more easily. Making them feel like they're not getting taken care of the right way, but they really are, too! Your feelings, emotions, mind & thinking, are altered a lot of times; and you're not thinking the same way you need to be.

Due to your Epilepsy & Seizures, too! That's just a normal response in people who suffer with these kinds of medical issues also? You never know when that's going to be worse either? Since you can't really predict when you're going to be having any of your episodes or seizures? They just happen when it's time for them to happen? That's something that's pretty much an unpredictable thing, and can't be helped with Epilepsy, too! It's not your fault though, because it's just part of the disease… That nobody can really do anything about, but try to understand a little bit better. That's all I do know about that, because it's easy to feel like it's your fault; and you know it's not. There's lots of things that Epilepsy affects, and one is how you feel a lot about yourself in general?

It can really make you feel terrible about yourself a lot, too! That's when you've got to grab a hold of yourself, and pull yourself, together? So, that you can do something that'll help make you not feel so bad. Since you don't want to let it control how you're feeling? Plus, you can't help, but feel the way you do… When you've had the seizures, too? They always generally make you feel very bad! One thing I've learned to do is find things I'm grateful for, and that's something that helps out a lot also. It's not really that hard to do, because we've all got things we're grateful for. Sometimes maybe it's just difficult for us to see them all, but there right there in front of our faces.

If we look close enough? We'll see them, and write them down! Plus, tell yourself some Positive Affirmations, because that'll help a lot, too! With building your self-esteem up some more, because if you're an Epileptic? I'm sure you probably struggle with this one a lot, because I really do. That's a very big one for me, too! I used to have a better self-esteem than what I do now? I keep trying to build it back up again, but sometimes it's not very easy to do. Things with my Epilepsy have really taken a toll on me, and have caused me, too many other issues. That cause it to be harder for me, but I keep going through life struggling more sometimes; but trying to keep my faith up.

Hoping that everything will improve, and get better. Not knowing whether or not? It all will or not, but trying to believe that I know no matter how hard things God's always there for me. That comforts me, and keeps me from giving up, too! Even when it feels so bad that I'd really like, too? Plus, I keep on believing in myself, and trying to succeed in the things I want to do. That's really important for me, because it matters so much to me, too! I set aside times when I'm praying, but nobody else knows what I'm doing? Except for God, and sometimes I'll go to him; and pray even more. When I need to do that more in order for me to feel better, because it does help also?

I still get afraid, frightened & scared, because I'm human... All humans do, because of things that's happening inside their lives & others, lives. That freak them out, but make things unstable inside their lives, too! It's actually pretty normal, and I had a friend one time... Who said, "I'd be worried about you... If you weren't scared? Especially since, that's a normal reaction... You should be, but don't get overwhelmed and let it take complete control of you." I haven't talked with her in a long time, but I've not forgotten all the things... That I've learned from her, and how much they've helped me?

I still use everything she taught me today in my life, and it also is something that I'll never forget... There was more than one lesson that she taught me, because we were close friends. She gave me a lot of support, strength, friendship, but also helped me in ways... That I can't share some things with you about. I will say that if it hadn't been for her coming into my life? I wouldn't be the person that I am today, and wouldn't have 18 years of Sobriety either. That's why we were so close of friends, together? God was the reason that she entered into my life, because he's the one... Who intervened in my life to change the path of self-destruction? That I'd been going down for so long, too!

So, I'm very grateful for that friend... I'll never forget her, or the things she taught me either. They play an important part of my everyday life, and make my life better. Even though sometimes things are going so wrong inside my life... That it doesn't feel like it was worth it? Except I know that's a lie, and not really true. Why? If it hadn't been worth it? Then some things wouldn't have ever happened that's been so wonderful! That's how I know?

That's why I'm really grateful for the changes that's made me a different person, too? Plus, it's probably also helped with my seizures & Epilepsy, too! It sure couldn't have hurt at all! Everyone has their own story to tell, and I've got mine. I encourage you to share yours sometime, too! With everybody around the World, because you never know… Who you might be able to help? It's something that's pretty powerful, and people pick up Books all the time to read. Especially when they're interested in what somebody's got to say? Or what kind of Book they're wanting to read?

Chapter 6. What's Next

I'm wondering what's next? Well I don't know, because I'm still dealing with all kinds of problems. Plus, I'm still dealing with my Epilepsy & Seizures, too! Right now though I can tell you that things aren't very good, because there's some serious issues that's risen. That's got me questioning whether or not? The medications has caused some problems? Or whether or not the Peripheral Neuropathy is what's causing some of the problems? I recently went to see my doctor, because I've been very sick… My body's been rejecting certain foods, beverages & medications, too! It's also been having some other problems, but nobody's been able to really figure out what's going on exactly?

I've been sick as a dog though, and it's not been very pleasant at all! Or if there's some other issues that's caused these other problems, and whether or not? I've got to have surgery or not? Nobody is sure yet? Possibly but that might not solve all my issues either, and I don't know what I'm going to do? I've not been able to eat a lot, but I've got a lot of things happening that's got no explanation right now… Making it very difficult to find out what's going on, because of multiple issues, too? I don't know if my body has its Auto-Immune System that's being attacked, too? That's also another possibility due to some of the problems that I'm having, but there's a whole bunch of things I've got to have checked out. It's possible, but that might not be it either; and finding out what's going on is a big problem for us all right now?

That's something that isn't known right now at the moment, but hopefully… We can find out soon! I just know that I've been really sick, and was told that some things like this could happen. If it was Neurologically related? That doesn't mean that it is either, but we haven't got a clue right now? Since nobody can find out what's wrong? On tests & labs, that's been done so far. They are just aware of the fact that I'm very sick, and can't really explain it much at the time being. It's really kept me from doing a lot of things lately that I've wanted to get done also. That's been very frustrating to me, too!

Especially with me trying to get all kinds of things completed and done, that I need to do. Plus, not just my work, but other things in my life in general. It's caused me to be behind in a lot of things, and to the point to where? I have had problems just getting up out of bed lately, because I've been so sick. We know though that I just had normal tests come back on all my lab tests that had to be done. One of them was for Organ Failure & Red Sickle-Cell Leukemia, but as of right now they are all ok. According to the lab tests anyway, unless it's just not showing up? We don't know, but realize that my doctor's got to keep a close eye on all this. It's very important, and I'm at high risk of it happening to me, too! So, what's next?

Me keeping up with all the things that I need to do… In order for me to get better? If I can keep getting some more improvements in my life to happen? If I can get the things taken care of that need to be, and they can help me? So, I'm not so sick, and am feeling better. Than what I am right now, but also maintaining my doctor appointments; and taking my medications every day & night, that I've got to take? Since they matter so much for my body to operate properly or better? Than what it would without them? If I didn't take them, and wasn't on them I'd be hurting a lot… Since it's something I have to have in order to survive & live.

Keep living my life, and trying to do the best that I can… With all the things that I want to accomplish. Before something actually doesn't allow me to do that anymore? When that time comes? I'll deal with it then, but not until then. I'm not ready to stop doing the things that I want to do. I'm not ready to die yet? I don't want, too! I want to keep living, because there's still a lot of things left for me to do… Before I go?

I want to keep trying to get better if I can? So, that I can do other things, too! Not just my work, but to do some things that I've not been able to do for a while… That are a lot of fun! At least to me they are, and some of them are some things… That I've done before, but was made to stop. I'd like to give that stuff another try, because I enjoyed doing those things. Like going Bowling, and having some fun with my Spouse, together. Meeting other people, but doing something that's physical & fun, at the same time… Where lots of people are having a good time, and enjoying themselves, too?

Plus, go doing some other things like going for walks, and enjoying Nature again. Since that's something I really used to enjoy doing a lot, but it's not as easy for me as… What it used to be, because of some of my Neurological Health Problems? Like my Peripheral Neuropathy & Fibromyalgia. Plus, my Heart Problems can often cause me to have some difficulty with walking now also. Depending on how far & weather conditions, too? Plus, the fact that I'm still not out of the woods with my seizures either… Except they're better now, but you've got to keep in mind. I could have them at any time, and really don't need to be out venturing alone either for my safety. I know that I don't want anything to happen to me, but my Spouse doesn't either; and if I was out alone that something possibly could?

For now inside my life all I can do? Is keep doing what I've been doing? Moving forward, and trying not to go backward. Since that's not the right spot I need to be at, but headed towards the future... Is right what I'm focused on? That's very important to me, too! Since my well-being is at my own best interest, but also some other people's inside my life, too! That really matters a lot, because that's what's going to help me the most? Instead of going backwards, and my seizures getting out of control again... Not being as good as what they are now, because that wouldn't be a real good thing for me at all?

Right now I feel like it's a blessing for me to be where I am at today inside my life, too! It truly is, because if it hadn't been for the right doctor's helping get me on track... They all know who they are, too? Then things might not have worked out to my best interest at all, and I wouldn't be getting any better. Needless to say, that I might not even be here. If it hadn't been for all their help? That's what has made a World of difference in my life, but I will not ever be completely seizure free. Why? I believe it's, because of the Epilepsy; and partly due to my Adopted Dad beating me in the head as a child. Using hammers & tire irons, all over my head & skull; that's caused me to have significant brain damage & bruising, that'll never go away!

How do I feel about that you might ask? I'm very resentful, angry, but I hate him! I hate him so much, because I feel like I was robbed of my life. That my life would've been so much different if he'd never mistreated me? If I'd not been his Adopted Child, and had came from a better family? That I could've had a better life maybe? That maybe I'd been loved, and not ever mistreated by anyone. Since he wasn't the only one, but I've got absolutely no forgiveness for that Monster! I hate him, because of everything about him! If he was dead?

I'd like to bring him back myself, and send him back to Hell where he belongs? Since I don't know… If he's alive or dead? I wish sometimes that he'd come try to find me, because I'd give him every ounce of anger I've inside of me for him. I've been keeping set to the side just for his sorry ass! Sorry, but that's how I really feel about him. I know somebody told me well you shouldn't ever apologize for… How you feel? That's true, but I don't want anyone getting offended; because of how I feel about my Adopted Dad? That's just the truth, and at least I'm being honest about it.

My feelings I own them, and I've every right to them also. Nobody else could say… How they'd feel in that kind of situation? Unless they've been through it, and know what it feels like? Then they might be able to understand where I'm coming from? I believe that it makes perfect since, because all you've got to do is think of the outcome of walking through that kind of pain. For the rest of your entire life, and not having very many people who actually understand what that's like? It's like being in a storm that's not going to end, and you want out so bad! That man was inside of the Military, but he was a rotten egg in my eyes; and he always will be!

I don't believe that his real life played a good part in his own life either, because he didn't have a very good home either; but him being inside the Military made him a hell of a lot meaner & crueler, to me! I do believe that everything in life isn't fair, but that shouldn't mean… Other's should be mean to you! I don't believe that people have the right to be mean to people, because they want, too. Except I know that this often happens, and sometimes there's nothing we can do about it. Except accept them for who they are, and not have anything to do with them? Sometimes staying away from those kinds of people is about all we can do. As long as we don't act on actions, and do something cruel & mean, back in return… That could hurt us or them & others, because we shouldn't do that. We can all do something, but that takes us doing it; and it's praying for them & walking away!

No matter how angry or upset, we are with them? We can always do that, and move forward instead of going backwards. That's important, because it'll make you feel better. Don't worry about it… If somebody calls you a coward? For walking away, because that person isn't as smart & wise, as they believe they are. If they were? Then they'd chosen to walk away & pray, too! I do believe that, because that's not always the easiest thing to do in life. Especially when some people don't believe they're wrong at all?

You know, and they do also. So, does God, too! You see I'm on a mission right now… Of healing, because I want to get better. That's what matters to me, and if I let what happened to me? All those years so long ago get in my way. I won't achieve or succeed in the things that I want to do, because I'm giving up on myself. Giving up on all the things that really matter, and what happened then? I can't change, but I can go forwards with my life in the right directions. Trying to make the best out of every situation that's good & bad, too! That's having choices & freedom, and not letting them win!

Being in control of your life, because you don't want someone else controlling it. I'm human though, and one thing I've learned… Is we all make mistakes, and nobody should ever be put up on a pedestal? If we do that? We've set ourselves up for a big disappointment, because they might let us down. That's just a fact, and something I had to learn the hard way, too! It's so true, because we can see so much good in a person; but then suddenly they'll let you down. When you need them the most maybe, too? Maybe they didn't mean to either, but that doesn't mean… That it didn't hurt?

Sometimes that just is something that's going to happen, and when it does? We can't stop it from happening, because it's not us that was doing it. Unless it was? Then we might have to go back, and say to somebody… That's not what we intended to happen, and we're sorry for what happened? To make amends, and try correcting our own mistakes. That's a valuable lesson, but we don't have to always make amends. When we can learn how to stop having to make them, because we've grown enough? To where we don't mess up so badly, and owe them to anyone anymore? That can really make you feel good, but being an Epileptic that's nearly impossible doing sometimes; because we can mess up a lot.

Especially over our mood getting out of control when we've had seizures? Making us a lot more hateful or crankier than normally, too! It's not impossible, but more difficult learning how to get control of it? Once we do it's so nice, and not so bad! It can make a difference in how we feel about ourselves, too? Since it can affect everything about yourself, and how you feel overall about everything inside your life also. Epilepsy & Seizures, are often that way… That's just a part of it, and learning how to deal with it all? It makes a lot of things unpleasant in life for you, too! That's another thing I don't like about being an Epileptic, but I do my best to deal with it.

My doctor recently asked, me if I wanted to go up another notch on my newest medication? I said, "No, because I'm comfortable where it's at? Since I'm on so much medicine, and I often am very groggy. Feeling overmedicated sometimes, too! I also didn't think that it'd make that much difference, because of what I've been told in the past?" So, he was fine with me not going up another notch, too! That made me feel better, because I really think that I don't need to do that also. Since I'm maxed out on one of my seizure medications, and the second seizure medication has caused me to be somewhat unhappy. Even though it's gotten me better seizure control with my seizures, and my other medication. It's got side-effects that are more uncomfortable than the other medication does, too!

One was the weight gain difference, and it doesn't make you feel very good about yourself. Except it's not the kind of weight that's easy to get off of you. When you're so limited at what you can do, because of your health problems? Plus, it's not like it really wants to come off either, and that's very depressing, too! I really would like to see all of my seizures disappear completely, but I don't think that increasing my medication is worth it? Why? I'm on so many different medications, and I'm at risk like anyone who has to take so many? Of having problems with Organ Failure, and nobody wants that to happen to them! You see these kinds of medications are extremely hard on the Liver & Kidneys, but also the rest of your Organs. Especially when they can cause them to shut down, but your body depends on the life saving benefits of the medications in order for you to survive.

That's the thing… You can't just stop the medications, because you're worried about that. If you did? Then you risk something actually terrible happening to you? So, you've got basically no choice, but take your medicine properly. So, you can live your life, and hope… That you're going to get better! Sometimes it takes more than one, and sometimes it takes… A whole bunch of them to work, too! It just depends I guess, on how stubborn your body is going to be?

Or how severe & bad, your Epilepsy & seizures; are, too? That seems to vary with everybody who has the disease also, and it's not generally the same for everyone either? Which makes every situation unique in itself, too! Especially since we're all different anyway, but we're all special, too! Just because somebody is an Epileptic they're often seen as an extra special person, too! Simply for the reason that they are special, but they've got a lot of special needs, too! Which makes them get more attention sometimes than some, but it's only for their best interest; because they might really need that. They require a lot more things than most people, too! Needing help with things sometimes, because of their problems; and having to have an extra hand to help them with things in their life. Just since they've got to have someone helping them more doesn't make them bad either!

Sometimes it makes them not be so independent as they'd like to be, because of their Epilepsy. That's when they need a lot more help, and might require more attention? Due to them not being able to do some things by themselves, because of their Epilepsy & Seizures. One big key factor is the fact: They could go into Epileptic Seizures, and not come out? Or start going into seizures, and need help immediately? Having something else happen during the seizures, too! That could cause them to die if they'd not had help at all? That's the truth, and it can even happen inside a bathtub or swimming pool. Or outside mowing the lawn & vehicle, too?

Plus, it's something that could happen while inside their home, too! Or it could happen somewhere while they're out also, and you're on a family trip? It doesn't matter, but they can happen anywhere... That's my point! It could happen to them if they were trying to operate any kinds of heavy machinery, too? That's another thing that could happen, and it really does make them feel uncomfortable inside their lives; because of them having Epilepsy. It's not a fun thing to have, and it doesn't make you feel very happy most of the time either. It's an uncalming thing to have to overcome, because it makes life so unmanageable at times, too! It's just something that happens, and it can't be prevented really. You don't have any control over that, because there's no way to control that when it occurs?

Most people who've got Epilepsy know that, too? Except a lot of people who don't have it? May not fully understand what this is really like? They've got no idea... How much it affects your life either? Unless you share with them about what happens to you, and what's going on with you also? Then they might have a better understanding. They also might have a better understanding if they're familiar with Epilepsy? Plus, what it does to a person, and the consequences of the disease itself, too? It helps having the right knowledge about something, and knowing the true facts about it a lot!

It also helps when you let others around you know what could happen to you? If you were to have seizures, and they're not familiar with the disease itself? So, that they can be prepared to help you... If it's necessary, too? Since you never know when you might have seizures, and they're going to happen? That way if they occur? They can do something to help you, and make sure... That you also don't hurt yourself or injure yourself during the seizures. Since that is something that can often happen, too! Plus, since you might not be able to give them a warning when they're coming you can help educate them on how to help you?

Unless there's a Nurse around? Then they'll already know what to do? Which is a very good thing, too! They can help you more than anyone, but there's lots of people that can help... Don't get me wrong. I'm just saying, because that's true! Sometimes it's better if there's a Nurse or Doctor around? That can help you when you're having the seizures, but that might not always be the situation that you're in? For them to be present when you're having Episodes of Epileptic Seizures? It's not always the case when they're around you is what I meant by that?

There's things that can be done... When a person is having seizures, and is an Epileptic? That can help them out a lot! They are as follows: Turn them over on their side right or left, and let them be able to move freely. In case they were to vomit or throw up? Don't stick anything inside of their mouth, because they could bite it or choke on the object? Plus, make sure they don't stop breathing, their heart doesn't stop beating, and they're not turning blue! Also make sure that they're conscious after the seizures, but if they've lost control of their bladder? Help them get up, because they're probably going to need help walking; and might be dizzy headed or faint?

Then maybe you could help them get themselves cleaned up, but also get some clean clothes on, too! Keep an eye on them, and make sure that they're going to be ok. Let them rest, but make sure they stay hydrated also. They might be very thirsty, and not as much hungry. Since seizures can also affect the appetite quiet a bit, and make you less hungry a lot. Usually they'll feel very tired, and just want to sleep. They might also have a very bad headache, because of the seizures happening. Needing a darker room to rest inside of, too! Make sure that they're going to be ok even while they're resting, because when a person is an Epileptic? You really don't want to take any chances on them not being ok?

Since they can have problems, and it result in death from the seizures, too! You don't know that they won't have some more sets or episodes, of seizures… After having the ones that they've already experienced either? Which could result in something else taking place with them also, and you really need to pay attention to what's going on with them? In case they need your help? They might count on you a whole lot more than you know, too! Since they've got no control over what's happening to them also? You might be all they've got to count on, too! So, don't take that for granted or them either? Plus, they more than likely feel the same way about you as you do them, too!

That you're as important as they are, and that it'd be awful! If anything bad happened either way? Since they care so much about you, and you do them also. Being an Epileptic can make you a very weird person sometimes, because you may not act as normal as others. Except there's nothing bad about that, because it's just a personality issue you're dealing with… That's different from most other people's would be, and they're not going to know. Why? You're acting the way you are unless they know you're an Epileptic? It also can be beneficial to you as well, because it can keep you safer. Since sometimes people just want to stay away from you, and they just don't understand; but that's not always a bad thing either!

Especially when they might not be such a good person to be around anyway? You just never know until you find out? I'd rather them stay away, and not be hurt… If that's how they are? Since I don't need that anyway, but neither do you! We all need to have love, hope, faith, and good people inside of our lives… That really do care about us, because that's so important! Plus, it's very hard to find sometimes! Then sometimes it's not, but sometimes… We don't even have to look that far, because it's right there in front of us the whole entire time; and we're just noticing it!

Chapter 7. Now

Today inside my life I've learned a lot about the disease of Epilepsy, and not just dealing with it myself. Also how some other people have learned to manage their problems, and deal with it, too? I've been educated more about things the proper way, because of better doctor's helping me to understand… What I needed to about Epilepsy? Also about how it's affected me, and the things that it's caused me to have more issues with… Concerning my health, too! I've learned a lot about the mood swings, but also the depression that goes along with it also. Plus, I've learned how to deal with the extra problems that it's caused me to struggle with in my life, because I've gotten multiple Neurological issues over my Epilepsy causing me more issues, too! It's been a real struggle, but has taken a lot of time to get things in order; and under control with my seizures. I had a lot of people that treated me who gave up on helping me get better?

I know and understand, the patience that it takes dealing with this kind of health issue also. It can be very tiresome, frustrating, difficult & unmanageable, at times. However that doesn't mean that it's not controllable at all? Since I've hope today, because my seizures are controlled better… Than what they have ever been in my entire life? They're happening less frequently, but I still have them. Except they're not quiet as bad now as they've always been. I don't have back to back sets all the time, and am not completely unmanageable; because of the medications that are helping me. That's what has made one big difference, but another is the doctor's who took the time to help me, too? Without their help I wouldn't be in the spot I'm at today, and be able to be having so much better seizure control over my Epilepsy.

It's really made a big difference in my life, and how I feel about myself, too? Especially since I felt so hopeless at one point, but I didn't give up searching for somebody... Who could actually help me the way I needed it? That could find the right combination of Epileptic Medications, and get me on the right track. To where I needed to be the whole time also, but that's not an always easy thing to do? Since the disease of Epilepsy can be so difficult sometimes in certain individuals, and maybe not so hard in others. It can become very overwhelming, too! Making you feel very upset, because you don't know what to do? Or what's going to happen next? Often I had thoughts of suicide, because I became so depressed over my seizures & side effects, from the medications, too!

That took a lot of time spending it with a Counselor who could help me? Work through the issues that I needed to get past, and move forward. There sure was a lot more there than I really expected to discuss, but it worked! Sometimes we have to do things we don't want, too? In order to get the full benefit, and get better. Not just physically, but also emotionally. Since there's things that don't just affect us physically, and will often affect us in lots of ways emotionally, too! That's just another part of it, and if anyone says? They've not felt that way I wouldn't believe them, because it can happen taking the medications; but it's not something that should be ignored or overlooked. It's important that if you feel that way?

You've addressed it with someone who can help & understand? Especially since it's not a real good area to be inside your life, and you should talk to somebody about it also. That's very important, because everyone matters. Everyone has got problems, but that doesn't mean... If you go to somebody? Telling them that you feel like committing suicide they won't help you, because I'm willing to bet they'll listen. Since it's not a game, and it's your life at stake. It's a matter of life & death, sometimes; because of you feeling the way you do after your seizures, too. It's also that way taking the medications, and anyone around you needs to be aware of the side effects that the medications are causing you. Plus, I'm pretty sure that they care, because they're in your life; and don't want anything to happen to you either?

Epilepsy doesn't just affect the brain, but it also affects the mind. It also affects the whole entire body, and not just your brain & mind; but also the heart, lungs, muscles, liver, kidneys, colon & stomach. Why? It controls the whole body, and has the power to cause your body to have muscle aches, pains, spasms, cramps & migraines. It can cause you to lose your appetite, and feel very sluggish. It can cause severe major mood swings & depression, but it can cause vision problems also. Plus, it can cause problems concentrating, focusing, completing tasks & functioning in general, too! It can make you almost immobile at times... When it's very bad, and your Epileptic Seizures aren't controlled very well by your treatments being given? It can also cause you to want to isolate, withdraw, and be suicidal.

That's why I mentioned that? I know from experience, and what I've had to deal with from my own problems with Epilepsy & Seizures? Being so bad, but causing me to feel so terrible, unworthy, unloved, or a burden. Since the problems caused from seizures affect everything inside your whole life… Making your life very unpredictable & unbearable at times, too! Plus, how much of it can make you feel so down, depressed & upset, about everything in your life, too! Causing you to be very emotional, and having a lot of emotional outbursts maybe at times, too! Sometimes it just gets the best of you, but that doesn't mean… You can't get past that, because you certainly can! I believe that if I can anyone else can, too?

I know that everyone has their own ways of coping, but I use God a lot… Leaning on him, and talking to him. Giving him my prayers, heartaches, concerns & problems, because I know… He's always there, but that I can talk to him about anything, too! I don't just talk to him in times of need, but all the time… When other people don't know what I'm doing? They really don't have, too! I'm just making a point. I use music a lot to help me cope, too! I also journal some, and I do other things to help me get through things also.

I've got some Positive Affirmations that I include in my life all the time, too! I also have other things that make me feel better like reading, drawing, singing, knitting. I've not knitted in a long time though. I've had a lot of other things to do, and take care of instead. I used to paint, too! I've not done that in a long time either. It's ok though, because it's not going to matter either way right now with things. I like candles, and used them a lot to help me relax & cope, with stress also. Plus, even though it might sound crazy, but isn't Bubbles are great! Just sitting outside, and blowing bubbles is a wonderful stress reliever, too!

A lot of people who suffer with Epilepsy? Understands what that's all about and means? Since it's something that can happen a lot, but takes time getting used, too! Who really needs some help dealing with their emotions, because of how the medication & Epilepsy? Can make them feel, too! It's ok to have those feelings, but please seek help somewhere without acting on them. If you can? I think that's in your own best interest, and you'd be happier if you did? I wouldn't want you to act out on those feelings of suicide either. If you had them, because there's nothing in life worth suicide?

I've heard from people in the past? That it was mind over matter, and that really made me angry. Since I didn't feel like they really understood at all. What I was going through, but that was it? They didn't, and other people who knew how to deal with my problems did? All it took was finding the right person or people, but having their help... With what I was going through to help me get through it all? It was mind over matter, too! Only it really didn't feel like it, but they're just feelings... That can be very scary, difficult handling & emotionally mindboggling, too!

There's absolutely nothing wrong with having help overcoming those awful feelings & emotions. Especially when you might not be able to get through it all by yourself, and you really need somebody? It's ok, and don't let anyone tell you that it's not ok to ask, for help? It's better than the outcome of not asking, for any help at all? Plus, it's the right thing to do! You want to be able to share your experience with somebody someday, too! I mean it's a pretty big deal, because you can help someone who needs it? Plus, I'm sure it's a great story or Book, that you can write about yourself; and share your strength, hope, experiences, but also how you've gotten through it, too? What are they going to do? Laugh at you, but that shouldn't matter; because I've been laughed at.

That didn't stop me, because I've learned how to laugh at myself; and my problems sometimes, too? Why? I got tired of having my feelings hurt, and it helped me get used to being the way I am. Without being hurt all the time by others, and them being very mean to me. Just because they didn't understand what I was going through? Plus, it taught me how to gain backbone... Dealing with some really mean people who just like making fun of other people, and being immature? That's what they are is immature for making fun of people? Who have health issues? So, what I'm an Epileptic?

I have seizures, and you think it's funny? Ha, ha... I guess, I'm you're big joke for the day. Well that doesn't hurt my feelings one bit. Laugh all you want, too! That's how I feel to all those people who don't understand? That's so immature, and haven't got a clue. What it's really like dealing with these kinds of problems? They're not that important to me, and I don't let them rent space... Inside of my head either!

So, I got hit in the head when I was a little kid a lot? By hammers & tire irons. Oh, well... I'm like a butterfly that got thumped over the head one, too many times. Ha, ha! You think that's funny do you? I don't care! Laugh at me all you want, too! That doesn't bother me, but it might you at some point. I guess, too bad... That it wasn't the person who thought it was so funny to begin with?

Oh, well that's how people are sometimes; but that's ok, too! I'm willing to bet that they're not laughing at me now. They're inside their own hell, and that's why? Life isn't always pretty! That serves them right. As far as I'm concerned, because it's not my fault! Sometimes people get exactly what they deserve? That was their fault, and I had nothing to do with that. So, they can't blame me for it, but I don't listen to them anymore. They're no longer inside of my life, because of how they treat people?

I've moved on, and I don't let them rent space inside of my life anymore either! Since that's all they wanted to do anyway, but sometimes we find out the hard way. How people really are? Sometimes not soon enough, because it takes longer for their true colors to come out; and they've been hiding behind a persona trying to fake who they really are? That's what happened in that particular situation, but the main thing is? I'm ok today, and better off knowing that they weren't a friend at all. True friends don't treat people that way, because a real friend is an honest person that cares about somebody through thick & thin, too! It never hurts to find out the truth about somebody, but it does hurt when we find out the truth sometimes? Especially if they've done something that hurts us & others, but has a major affect on our lives, too?

Being an Epileptic I weed out the bad people in my life, and keep safe boundaries. I don't need those kinds of people inside my life, because they might create more issues for me. That's detrimental to my health, too! Which I don't want either, because I'm still working on healing & my journey, too! Getting better down the path that I've been trudging along on, and hoping that more things will improve also. Since I really need them, too! I keep a lot of people out sometimes, but I feel safer that way. Plus, it's very difficult for me to trust others also. I let people in very slowly over a period of time, but it takes a while usually for me to know… If I can really trust them or not?

Sometimes I can tell immediately, because of the nature of that person's attitude & personality? I have a thing about this normally that also helps me, and that's called an Aura… It's a psychic capability that helps me know in some cases if I can trust somebody or not, too? It's a feeling that's very familiar to me, and alerts me right away. If I can't, too? It's very strong, and will often frighten me to death! When I feel it, because it reminds me of people from my childhood? When I feel that? I'll stay away quick, too! I have an extra sense where I know things others don't, but it's not a bad thing?

Often a lot of the times Epileptics will keep a lot of things to themselves, because of being afraid… To share things with other people, and not let people get very close to them. Feeling like they couldn't handle being around them. If they knew the truth about what they were struggling with? Or if they'd be bothered by them being an Epileptic? Or if it's, too much for someone else to deal with? Since it's a very serious condition, and needs a lot of care handling, too! Plus, it requires a lot more attention in most cases than a lot of things do. Simply for the fact that something could happen at any time, but you're not sure when? Plus, there's all kinds of things that can be embarrassing to deal with, too!

That's just another part of having Epilepsy, but most of the time people won't openly talk about this. Except with those that's around them the most, because they know? That they'll understand. Where others might not? Unless it's your doctor? They will also usually understand, but they're usually pretty used to dealing with these kinds of issues. When it comes to dealing with so many patients who have Epilepsy? So, they don't judge & look down on you, because of it either. Plus, there's other people who need to know? How to deal with you in times of crisis, too?

Since you've got Epilepsy, because it'll help them know what's going on better with you; and that might what's happened? Especially after your seizures, because you might not be acting like yourself at all? Plus, there's been a numerous amount of occasions… When you'd thought I was drunk? Except that wasn't it, because of my seizures being so bad… I seemed like I was drunk, because of how I was acting? I couldn't even hardly walk straight, because I was so dizzy headed; and was having trouble with my eyes, body & mobility, too! Plus, I was having difficulty talking, and couldn't speak hardly at all… To where anyone could understand me? I was totally disoriented, too!

It wasn't my fault, but due to my seizure activity... Plus, what they'd done to me afterwards, too? There wasn't anything that I could do about that either, because it was... What it was? Epileptic Seizures & Episodes, causing me to not act the way I normally did. That's pretty much all it was, too! After resting, and getting myself to feeling better? The best that I could... I was sort of able to return back to kind of normal. Normal as to what's normal for me?

That's different for everyone who has Epilepsy, too? Remember, I told you we all have similar symptoms? Maybe not all the same at once, but sometimes we can relate to others... By knowing that we've had all the symptoms at one point or another? They range & vary, in all kinds of different ways, too! Coming from multiple symptoms, and just a few. Like three or four, at a time? Plus, they can multiply sometimes by seven or eight, too! Epilepsy has many complications & problems, but the person(s) dealing with it struggle the most. That's just a true hard fact about how it affects you & others, inside your life?

It's a hard task for anyone to handle, but also get a grip on. Except it can be done! If you're willing to fight against it? Keep fighting against it, and not let it win! Not give it the power that it wants, and the control over your life... It's constantly trying to take away from you! That's what it wants, but that doesn't mean you're defeated by no means? Especially since you can gain the strength you need from deep within, but also from taking the medications your doctor gives you. Plus, by dealing with what you need, too? Inside of counseling, if necessary? You can build on your own inner strength, and keep getting stronger to overpower it!

Plus, believe that God will help you get through it, too! That's where you'll even get more strength? To help you gain better control over your Epilepsy, and to make yourself feel better, too! Plus, it'll help you build your self-esteem, hope, confidence & belief in yourself more. It'll give you encouragement to get through so much more... Than just your Epilepsy, too! You can start with that, and then take on bigger things... That's in your way that might be a struggle, but also overcome them also. I'm going through a lot of things right now in my life, and it's not easy to do. I'm struggling, but I'm trying to keep that same attitude I've had about my Epilepsy; and get through it all.

Except I'm very frightened, but I guess that's ok. It feels hopeless, but I know it's not. Plus, I don't know what's going to happen next? It's got me upset, and also pretty freaked out! Also I'm not sure what's going to be done about it? So, I'm worried, too! I've faith, but that doesn't mean that I'm not scared. I also don't know if it's something that could be Neurologically related either? I've got no idea, because right now... Nobody's sure exactly what's going on with me?

I know that having Epilepsy can be a real unpleasant thing, but there's a lot of things... To help you get through it also, and now they've got a lot more ways. Of handling it than what they used to have a long time ago, too? To help you better understand what's going on with you also, but also educate you in more ways... That's beneficially going to help you down your road of recovery fighting with seizures & Epilepsy, too! Plus, there's a lot more things that they can do now, too! It just depends on what's best for you? What they believe will help you? Plus, what works for you, because what works for you might not for someone else? It varies for each individual who's fighting the disease of Epilepsy, and isn't the same for everyone.

I wish that there was a cure for having Epilepsy, but there's not! It's something they don't have a cure for, but they can manage it better now. Than what they every could in the past? There's a lot of better medications now a days... Than what they used to have, too? They cost a lot of money, but sometimes you can get help getting them. If not your doctor will figure out something that they can do for you, too! So, never give up hope on that!!! It's important to understand that just, because there's no cure for Epilepsy doesn't mean... You can't get better, and improve with your seizure activity & Epilepsy?

I'm living proof that it can happen, and I'm sure I'm not alone! Here's an example... About five or six years ago, I was told that I wasn't ever going to get better! That my seizures were always going to stay as bad as what they were? Well since last year, I've been able to improve a lot! I'm working now, and doing what I've always wanted to do, too! Nobody thought I was going to get better, but all it took? Was the proper medical attention & medications, for me to get on the right track. Then major things started happening inside my life that turned my whole World around in a different direction! I still have seizures, but I'm doing much better now; and they don't happen all the time either!

Which makes my life a little bit better, and I say only a little bit; because I've still got a whole bunch of problems. That I've got to handle daily, but I'm doing the best that I can to manage everything to the best of my ability. That's something that matters to me, too! Plus, it means a lot... Knowing where I've come from, and to the point I'm at now in my life? Since all the problems that my Epilepsy, and seizures has caused me, too! Keeping me from doing so many things inside of my life that I really wanted to do, too! Making me so unfunctional & zombie; out a lot also most of the time. Since they made me feel so groggy, and I could barely function at all or get out of bed? All I could do, but felt like doing most was sleeping over them.

Or I was to upset & distraught, to get very much of anything done? That I really wanted to do, because of how bad the seizures had made me feel afterwards? Putting me in a deeper state of dark depression, and I felt like my whole World... Was tumbling down, and crashing on top of me! Making me feel so small & weak, because of how they were affecting my body? Plus, how they made me feel all, together? Since they never make you feel all that great? I've never heard from anybody who has Epilepsy? "Oh, I feel great!" After having their seizures, and trying to recover from them?

That's just how bad? Epilepsy can really make a person feel, because it doesn't make you feel very good at all! No matter when the seizures are happening? You can't stop it, and basically you've just got to let them... Ride out their course, until they're finished? Waiting can be a hard one, too! Since you don't know how long it's going to take? Before you're feeling better, because the recovery time afterwards can also vary... Every time you have your episodes, too! It's probably not the same every time, because mine wasn't.

It still isn't either, but it's sometimes better; but sometimes not as good also. Sometimes I've got severe chest pains to deal with, because of my seizures. Needing to take some other medications to help me deal with that, because of my Epilepsy & Seizures; being what's caused those problems to develop to begin with? I do what I need, too? In order for me to take care of myself, because I know... How important that is, too? Plus, I've got to take care of me... Especially if I want to be around here for a while, and not have anything happen to me? Also so I can be here for my Spouse & Pets, too! Plus, maybe so I can help someone else, too!

That's what I'd like to be able to do with this, too? Is help others by sharing my experience, strength & hope, with what I've been through? On my own journey with having Epilepsy, and how it's affected me & others, inside of my life? Plus, how things have been able to give me something to look forward, too? Since everyone said, "I didn't have any hope before, because they never saw me getting better. Or had given up on me completely?" They were all wrong, and I'm better! I'm able to do the impossible now that they said, I wouldn't be able to do before, too! That really makes me feel good, because I'd really tried doing that multiple times before in my life, too! Plus, it just goes to show that they're not God, and don't have the right to say nobody will get better either!

Chapter 8. The Future

I don't know what the future holds? About my Epilepsy &
seizures, but I do know… That if I continue taking my
medications, and keep my doctor appointments? That they will
be about as good as they're going to be. Since they'll never
completely stop! Except they're much better now than what
they've ever been in my life? So, if I keep going down the path
I'm on? Maybe some other things will get better, too! Maybe
some other things will also improve over time, but I'm not sure
if that'll happen? That's what I want to happen though, because I
want to feel better; and keep getting better.

As much as I possibly can? I also guess, that's not entirely up
to me… Whether or not? I continue to get a lot better, but I can
do what I can to maybe help? By doing the best I can to take care
of myself, and sometimes that might mean… Slowing down
some, too! I really don't like doing that, but there's sometimes I
don't have very much choice in that matter. I have, too! In order
for me to feel better sometimes, and that's just how it is? It's not
that I like it, but I have to do what's best for me?

Sometimes we have to do things that we don't like doing,
because that's what's best for us? Sometimes that means
stopping for a little bit… From whatever you're doing, and
taking a break? A breather or rest period, like a time-out for
yourself. Until you're feeling better, and then you can get back
to what you want to do? That makes sense doesn't it? I believe
so, because in a lot of situations… There's times like these when
things are, too difficult for us? When we need a break? To help
us get back to where we were at?

When we were feeling better, and we'll be fine doing that, too? It's not the end of the World if we've got to take some time out for ourselves, and step away from things a bit? Sometimes that's just life, because it can get the better of us. Making us feel bad, and we need to take a step back. That doesn't mean we've got to quit doing things we enjoy? It just is like a short pause, because we need a break... Stopping time for a little while, and putting things on stand still mode. I often have to do this a lot sometimes, but I try getting back to things... As fast as I can, because I really don't like having to do this at all! Plus, my health causes me to have to do this with all sorts of things I'd rather be doing; but that's life sometimes.

Life isn't fair, but that's just how it is? That doesn't mean we've got to always like it either. Just accept it, and move on... There's nothing else you can really do about it either except that. If you don't, and let it get to you? Then you're going to regret it, because you'll be in a World of hurt. That's not going to help make you feel any better about anything at all? Why? It's just going to bring you down more, and make you feel worse about your situation. Plus, get you all bummed out, too!

It might even cause your seizures to worsen, too? That's always possible, because stress has a big role in Epilepsy, too! As well as sleep patterns, too! You've got to get the right amount of sleep for yourself... When you're an Epileptic? That varies for everyone who has the disease, too! Since nobody is exactly the same, and some people might need... Lots more rest than others do, too! Just deal with it! They say, but that's so far easier said, than done!!!

Sometimes it's not always that simple, but that's what they don't understand? I'm right about that, but don't worry about it... Just overlook them, and try to handle things the best that you can. That's about all you can do? If you don't handle it well at first? Then keep trying, until you do get better? Sometimes that takes a whole lot of time, too! A lot of mistakes, I'm sorry's, and oh I didn't mean it! Please, forgive me... I won't do it again, but you really mean it.

Then when your seizures happen? It happens again, but don't give up. It'll get easier to deal with in time, and that's what we've got to learn? Time is a biggie on Epilepsy, because sometimes it makes you feel like you're doing time in a way. It's a life sentence having seizures & Epilepsy, because it's out of your control; and causes so many problems. It's almost like oh, my goodness... I've got this to deal with the rest of my freaking life? Are you freaking kidding me? It's so overwhelming, and can be so aggravating, too! Plus, it's like oh no, not again!

It can make you feel that way, because even though it's not the same thing as a life sentence... It's a life sentence dealing with a medical issue that's superbad! Trying to cope with, and deal with all by yourself. That causes severe major problems, and needs lots of medical expertise, too! Since it's not something that's curable, because it'll never just disappear. If it did? That would be wonderful, but that's not how it happens unfortunately? Once you've got it you're stuck with it, and everything that occurs with having Epilepsy, too! It's something that's life changing, but something that's a disability. You've got to learn how to deal with, and treat with doctors who know what they're doing?

Disabilities aren't always easy to deal with, but a lot of people... Don't understand what it is like dealing with those problems? Unless they're familiar with them? Or they've got an idea... As to what you're going through? Maybe they know someone who's got the problem? Or some other kind of disability? Any kind of disability can be hard to handle, and be very aggravating & frustrating; to deal with also. Not just having Epilepsy, but all disabilities are a struggle. Nobody is exempt when it comes to having disabilities, because they can happen to anybody, too?

I've learned in my lifetime... That some people think they are exempt from ever having any kinds of disabilities happen to them? That's not true though, because nobody has the say over what's going to happen to them? Sometimes things happen, and we least expect it, too! That's when the tough gets going, and the tough becomes you getting stronger? Or you can give up? Letting it get you down, and overpower you completely... Sometimes it's not a matter of you letting it overpower you or you giving up either? It takes control, and does whatever it's going to do; because it's not going to give your body a chance? That's just what does happen sometimes, but there's not anything we can do about it then?

Having Epilepsy is like that, too! Sometimes a lot of people end up dying over it, and there's nothing that could be done... To stop it from happening? Especially if it happened while they were sleeping? Plus, nobody knew about it, and nobody was around to know what'd happened to them? The thing called SUDEP is a true thing, and that's sudden death with Epileptic Seizures. It can kill a person when this happens? It's usually when someone is sleeping, and goes into Epileptic Seizures; and they don't come out of them? They end up dying, but there's nobody that catches what's happening at that particular moment? Often it happens so quick, and fast that the person dies instantly, too!

When everything seems ok, but the person isn't being watched? Sometimes this can occur, too! It can often make others feel responsible, but it's not their fault. There's nothing they could've done to stop it, but sometimes people can't be around all the time. To make sure that somebody is going to be ok, and that's not their fault either. Sometimes things just happen, but we have no idea... What we could've done we think? To ourselves to help that person, and sometimes you couldn't do anymore than... What you'd already done? Checked on them, and they seemed ok.

So, you left them alone to sleep, and figured that they'd be ok. That's not your fault, because when something like this happens it's fate? It's their time to go, and God said, so... That doesn't mean it's not going to hurt. It's just his way of taking them out the most peaceful way in their sleep, I guess. So, they're not suffering anymore! That's what I believe? Since sometimes a lot of people do go about struggling with these problems & suffering, a whole lot, too! It can be that devastating & hard, to face the facts about having this kind of disease called Epilepsy. We're all miracles, because we're trying to cope with something that's so difficult; but nearly feels impossible overcoming at times, too!

When the body can't fight against them anymore? Bad things usually do happen, but there's nothing... That we can do about that very much either. Except what we've been doing? Taking your medications, and keeping up with your doctor appointments... The best that you can, and doing your best to take care of yourself, too! That's about all you can do, but sometimes others might need to help you also. That's sometimes the case, but don't worry about it! You need it, and if they didn't care they wouldn't be helping you? When you need somebody to help look after you?

I do know that dealing with this problem can be a real struggle, and it varies all the time... About how you feel? Especially when you've had seizures, but they make you feel so terrible? All you can do is try to get through it that moment, and take it easy. Give yourself some slack, but credit also... Since you're going to need, too! When the episodes occur things are more difficult for most people? Who're struggling with Epilepsy, and trying to fight against the disease itself, too! It's just a part of it, but don't let it get you down one bit; because you don't deserve to let it get the best of you! It's something that you learn to manage in time & often, it takes more time than immediately being able to fully gain control over it, too!

Plus, it's not something that's easy for everyone to get a grip on, but it's not impossible to manage over some time. Even when you're going to the doctor, and taking medications? You still have to usually find ways of dealing with it, because the seizures don't just disappear! That's the thing that everyone needs to understand, but it's great... If they do for some individuals, because I know that can happen, too? It just doesn't happen that way for everyone, and that's often disappointing. That's the thing about everyone being different, but not having the same experiences, too! No matter how hard the journey gets don't give up, because it's worth the fight? To overcome the Epilepsy & Seizures, as much as you can; but also to get better. Plus, you want to be well, and not as in bad shape as you are at that moment; because you want to heal?

I know that I did, and I still do… I also know that my
seizures won't completely go away, but that's not the end of the
World. Just because they won't get anymore better than what
they are now? Since I've been able to come so far along away of
a journey that nobody… Thought was ever going to be possible
for me to do? I've been able to heal & improve, because of the
right doses of combinations; and doctor's with my care dealing
with my Epilepsy. It also did help me when I went to intensive,
therapeutic, gut wrenching, Counseling before? That helped me
get to where I'm at today inside my life? I've come a long ways
from where I used to be at, too! I'm really glad, happy, excited &
pleased, over that also.

The road that I've traveled down dealing with this, and many
other things inside my life… Hasn't been a pleasant one, but it's
been a very rocky road! That I'm not ungrateful for at all,
because there was a reason I believe… That I had to go down a
different trail, and had so many obstacles in my way? Before I
could make it to where I'm at today? Except it was worth every
bit of pain, tears, sadness, complications & courage, I could find
within side myself to do it, too! I wouldn't want to do it all over
again, but I also at the same time… Don't regret any of it either,
because I'm right where I need to be now? That's important for
me to remember, too! That also makes this a lot more
meaningful to me, too!

Since it seems to me that a lot of things helped me… To be able to learn more about things. That I might not have been able, too! If it hadn't been for my very own experiences with dealing with multiple issues & complications? It doesn't really matter that I suffered a severe brain injury either, because of Epilepsy running in my family. Since I ended up having it before the brain injury, but I'm pretty sure… That didn't help me in any way either, because it made my problems harder to find ways in getting better control of them? In order to try to stop my seizures as much as they possibly could, too? After looking my whole life for the right things to help me get better? They were finally able to find some things that would work for me, and help me get better?

That was very important for me, too! Especially when a lot of people who were doctor's before? Had given up any hope of me ever getting better at all. Since they felt like it was an impossibility, but it wasn't! It was just that they didn't have the answers or solutions, because they weren't trying hard enough? That's what the real problem was there, and it's a fact… That often does happen to people. Who suffer with Epilepsy, too? Sometimes doctor's don't have the same education, tools, or experience… That other's do, and don't know exactly how to help some patients as well as others?

Except that doesn't mean they can't help other patients, but they might not be as equipped to deal with your own personal needs. That's just sometimes something that happens, but you can't stop looking for the right person to help you! They're out there somewhere, and you've got to find them. Sometimes some Insurances make that difficult, too! I know, but that's not your fault either. Just keep looking, because somebody will be able to help that does accept your healthcare Insurance. Hopefully they really can help you, too! I know that really does make a difference, and how aggravating it can be? To be able to succeed in that goal, because it's like a big accomplishment taking place inside your life. When that actually does happen, and you can start on the right path to healing with your Epilepsy?

Plus, it's something that will brighten you up a lot, too! It helps you feel better mentally also, because now you know... That you don't have to worry as much maybe? Maybe that you're going to start getting better, and making some major improvements? Sometimes those major improvements don't happen right away, but they'll come in time. Don't worry about it, because you've got to let your body... Have the time it needs in order for you to begin healing? Once your doctor can get you on the right track, but having you taking the proper medications, too! That's another important factor, because it's so true... Without that you can't get any better, and I believe everyone knows that who suffers with Epilepsy & deals; with it, too?

I don't have any comparisons for anyone, because I don't believe that you can compare Epilepsy... To any other problems, but I know that some things go hand in hand. They can feel very similar, because you might have some other issues... Caused from having Epilepsy, and they're something else you've got to learn how to handle, too? Like severe depression, and other Neurological Health Issues. That's often the case in a lot of situations, but it doesn't help sometimes... Since it can make things harder for others to understand. What's really going on with you? Since they might not know how to deal with your problems, and aren't familiar with what you're coping with? Sometimes the people around you can help with that, but not in every situation do they want, too?

It's not always the best thing to do, but in some situations it might be? It depends on who the other people are, and what's happening at the time? Don't worry about it, because you don't have to explain yourself to everyone. Keep them wondering, and move on... Ignore them, because you've got enough of your own problems to deal with. I wouldn't really waste my time much, because they don't understand... What's happening with me all the time? Maybe they really wouldn't care either? I don't really care if they do or not? Not my problem, because I just want to be left alone; and not bullied by others!

Sometimes people are just like that, and they don't know... How to really treat others? Don't worry about them, but take care of yourself. You're more important to be more concerned with what's going on with you? Instead of dealing with all their nonsense. Everybody doesn't react the same way thankfully, because everyone's not mean. Plus, everybody doesn't have the same kind of understanding... About certain things, but that's ok, because you don't need their approval. Since we're all made up differently genetically that helps, too! Make us our own person, and be more unique than others.

Just going through the flow sometimes can be the trick… To get us to our next, step to help move us past an obstacle that's standing in our way? Sometimes that'll give us that extra incentive that we need, too! There's lots of times I know… That I really needed that extra push, because things were getting to me so badly. Whatever it takes, I guess? That's going to be different for everyone, too! Since we've got to all find our own way of dealing with things, but getting through things. In order for us to feel better, and handle situations that can be devastating to deal with at times? It's going to be ok, because you can do it!

It's often a thing that can cause us a lot of disappointment at times, too! Since we've got more to cope with normally than most people… Why? We're a little bit different, because we've got a disease called Epilepsy. That causes things inside of our lives to be topsy-turvy a lot, too! Especially when things are very early on, and it's not something? That we know very much about, but we're just getting started learning all we can about having Epilepsy. Plus, all the problems that go along with it, too! That can make our life so difficult & unmanageable, also except we know there's hope. We've just got to get to that point to where we're doing much better, and have been able to successfully gain some seizure control?

That really helps us out a whole bunch, too! We know that we can make it there to that point, too! It just might take a little bit more time… Than what we wanted it to at first? It's ok if it does, too? Everyone has got a different journey that they all have to take… Walking through life having the disease of Epilepsy, and learning how to manage it inside their life also? It's not at all impossible for us to be able to prove everybody wrong, and do things… They said, we couldn't do before! Since we've got our own decisions in our care & treatment, but also we have the power to choose to make them wrong; and not let them win!

Plus, we might show them that we're stronger than they think we are, too! Which can be very powerful without saying the least, because that inner strength... Is a thing of beauty for all of us that we've got, too! Especially when we let it shine, and come out for everyone to see it? It's a great thing, because we know... What we've had to deal with? Plus, how we've managed to get through it, too? It's also something that nobody can ever take away from us, because we own that inner strength & beauty. Plus, it's something that really makes us feel pretty good & confident, about ourselves, too! Just for the simple fact that it causes us to feel a little bit extra special, and we know already that we are also.

It also makes us feel like we've got some control, and some power over our Epilepsy. Since we actually do a little bit, but maybe not when we're going to have our seizures? Or we might not be able to predict when they'll occur? Only we know that we're not feeling so good... For a specific reason, because we know they're coming! That's how Epilepsy does work, too? Since it has more control over that part, and your body... Than you want it to have, but sometimes that can be prevented? Since that's just a part of the instability with having Epilepsy. Especially when they override everything else that you're trying to do?

When we've got more stability with our seizures and control, of them? We feel better not just physically, but also emotionally & Spiritually, too! Since it can affect everything about us, and inside of our lives, too! That's just another part of it also that's often hard to deal with, but something that's learned... How to achieve coping with it? That doesn't mean that it's easy to do, but it's something that can take lots of patience & time! Doing things inside your daily life... Will help you to better achieve accomplishment in that goal, too? I know from my own experiences, because I had to learn how to do it? It's still a battle sometimes, but I can bounce back quicker now!

I'm really very glad about that, too! It makes me feel pretty good about myself today, and how much things have changed? Even though there's still a ton of issues that I've got to deal with? I do the best that I can, but then go on. Without giving up, and sometimes it's hard; because I feel like doing just that. When things get so bad, and are out of my control? I'm having a very difficult time dealing with everything, and it all seems hopeless again. Only something inside of me won't let me give up, because I've never been that way? Something inside me pushes me past that point, but it's not just inner strength; because it's also God. I give him all the credit for that, because it's true!

I am saddened to know... How many people actually die from having this disease of Epilepsy, too? It happens more often than not, and not many people will talk about that part of it. Why? I believe that it's, because it's so personal... It's also a very bad thing, and way to die. I'm blessed & grateful, that I'm still alive. I know how slim the chances have been where I almost didn't make it, because of my episodes of Epileptic Seizures? How close that I had to be resuscitated a numerous amount of times, too? That I wasn't breathing, and my heart had completely stopped.

I was blue in the face, but drooling... I'd lost all control of my body fluids, because of what had happened to me? It's not funny, because that's the facts about what can happen to an Epileptic? I'm not ashamed about it anymore, because I had people make fun of me. I don't care, because they didn't know what was wrong? They were to immature to understand what'd happened, and were stupid? Since they were making fun of somebody who was almost dead? That's complete ignorance, in my opinion! It's something that's very sad, and people should have respect for other's... About having these kinds of problems, too!

Epilepsy is for real, and it's a very serious condition that kills people. It doesn't care who you are? Or who it takes either, because it's got no boundaries? When it comes to ending people's lives, and causing them to die? Or affecting them, but causing them to struggle all the time... Getting through life, and trying to achieve things. That they really want to do? Except due to having Epilepsy it tries to make that nearly impossible. Only thing that Epilepsy does care about... Is taking total control of somebody who has to live with? Plus, how it affects other's inside of their lives, too?

Chapter 9. Attitude

Everyone who's got Epilepsy will have different attitudes… That can change like the wind, too! Since their moods never going to be the same all the time, because of how Epilepsy affects them? It'll make them be a different person than what they normally are sometimes? That's just part of it, too! I know from my own experiences… How often that has happened to me, because of my seizures? They can make you become very emotional, unstable, moody & irritable. They can make you get depressed, suicidal, or angry? Plus, they can cause you to feel very unlike yourself, too!

They can make you very withdrawn, silent, and cause you to be in your own little World, too! Also they can cause you to be agitated, because of you having the seizures. To have to deal with again, and knowing how frustrating that is? They also will cause you to feel sluggish, and make you feel upset about… Things that you might not normally be upset about, too! They can change you the second they happen, because that's what seizures & Epilepsy, does? That's just part of having Epilepsy, and trying to cope with it also. Sometimes they can cause you to be extremely hyper, too! Or make you go just absolutely bonkers, and become very high-strung, too? You won't react the same way that others will either most of the time, because we're all different; but that can happen to make your attitude change a lot.

A person who's got the disease of Epilepsy? Has many different kinds of attitudes mostly, too! Since they're battling something that changes them in so many different ways all the time. It does make sense, because it's not something that's easy to deal with... At the same time, and it causes you to not be the person you normally are, too! Just for the fact, that it can cause so many disturbances... Inside of your body, mind & emotional well-being, too! Plus, how it affects you physically & Spiritually, too? It'd be a lot different if it only changed certain parts of things about you? Except that's not what happens to somebody who has Epilepsy?

I've had to learn how to deal with all kinds of different attitude problems, because of my seizures & Epilepsy? It's not been something that was easy to do, and it took a lot of hard work... On myself, personality, attitude, health problems & medications, to help treat my Epilepsy correctly, too! Plus, it took a long, term of extensive out-patient care with a great Counselor... Who helped me get my life on track? Working through things that I needed, too! Plus, dealing with issues of my Epilepsy, too! Which was a really neat thing, because it's helped me in a lot of ways. I also had a support group dealing with other issues that was very beneficial to me, too! Which really worked out great inside of my life, because I had some other things that I had to take care of to get well also.

Attitudes & personalities, kind of go hand in hand also... Especially when you're dealing with these kinds of particular issues? Anybody who's got Epilepsy knows that, too? Since they've got to deal with these issues the most, and learn how to get a better handle on it all? It makes life harder, but it can also be a good learning experience. Since there's so many things that's pretty cool about how the brain & body, work? That you can also find out about... When you're dealing with Epilepsy? Trying to get your seizures on better track, and gain some control over them also. There's really a lot of things for you to learn when battling Epilepsy & Seizures?

Guess what? Having a positive attitude isn't the easiest thing to do. When you're dealing with Epilepsy? That's not a shocker to anyone who suffers from having the disease, but it's to other's? Since they don't always understand what it's like? Being a person who is struggling with having Epilepsy? Having a positive attitude the best you can… While trying to deal with it? Will actually help benefit you in the long run, because that kind of attitude… Will help you reach your goals of better care, treatment, control, and getting better.

Plus, it helps you with your healing process & recovery, handling the problems from your Epilepsy, too! So, if you've got a whole bunch of attitudes to deal with? Don't worry about it, but try to make sure… That you can get a handle on them, and not let them get out of control also? They can really be a big problem for an Epileptic, and sometimes for others, too! That doesn't mean that it's ok… To use that as an excuse, but try to take advantage of others. Just since you're having difficulty coping, and you've had seizures; because they make you more emotional & moodier? Just do the best that you can to make sure that you don't hurt others, because of having Epilepsy. When you have your episodes?

If you mess up? Try to correct the problem, and make amends as quick as you can. When you're feeling better, because there's no point in doing it immediately? If you might have some more right afterwards? The previous ones you had, but you should always try to fix your mistakes. I feel that's very important sharing, because I know… How easy it is to make those mistakes, but also people might not be so willing to admit the truth about it either? It does happen, and we don't generally mean for it, too! That's the thing, but we've got to gain control over our attitudes, too! So, people don't get the wrong idea about us, and just think we're a really uncaring individual that's mean or a bully?

I've shared a lot of things inside of here straight from the heart, but I believe you'll understand why? After going through these things yourself? If you're the one reading this, and you've got this disease of Epilepsy? The reason I did was, because I felt like the more experience, strength, hope & things, that I've dealt with… Might actually help others, too! Who have Epilepsy? Or somebody that knows somebody with Epilepsy? Or maybe someone who just wanted to read this, and find out… What it's all about? That's ok, too!

Being educated about it, but having knowledge on what it's like having Epilepsy? Is a really good thing, too! Especially if you don't have it? Or you're new to having it, and don't know what's going to happen in your life; because of it? The more people do know about it… The more they can help others, too! Plus, the more familiar they are with it, and understand? The better they can be towards a person struggling with it also. Maybe be their friend, and not judge them… Over them having Epilepsy, and being afraid of them.

Since they didn't have an understanding before, but they do now! That does generally help in a lot of situations, because you never know? When you could really help a person? Or meet somebody who has something like Epilepsy? That really is a pretty neat, cool, individual, too! They've just got some extra complicated problems in life to handle, and things are a lot more extreme to them also. That doesn't make them a bad person, but the disease is a bad thing… Except it can be taken with a grain of salt, too! Since you can do things to help yourself, too! Not letting it have the best of you, and take over your attitude & personality.

I encourage you... If you're the one reading this? Who has got Epilepsy? To be as informed with the correct information from your doctor that you can be... About having Epilepsy, and all the things that they can do to help you. Remember that it's not something that's got a cure, and maybe someday... They'll find one, but until then? We've got some really great tools the doctors can use to treat the disease. Some things I disagree with, but that's due to my own experiences... Like the VNS Implants, because I know what they can do to a person?

I know how many problems they can cause, and that they're not a cure? Like a lot of people want to say, but believe they are a great thing. I don't have that attitude about them, because I know what they've done to me & others, too? I believe that the VNS Implants are very bad medicine to use, and there's other medicines that can be used... Like the old-fashioned medicines you have to take orally, and maybe you don't like it? Except it's worth doing that, and saving your life instead of the alternative? Not everyone gets that chance, because they end up dying from having Epilepsy & Seizures, anyway! It's not fair, but that's what happens sometimes with Epilepsy? I don't believe that we should ever take life for granted, because of this. Plus we never know how much time we've got on Earth?

We're not promised anything, and that goes for another tomorrow, too! So, live your life to the best that you can, but also do something... That maybe will make you feel good, too! Help out someone else, because they'll really appreciate that a lot... I'm pretty sure about that, and you don't have to let everyone know. What you did either? Keep it between you & them, because that means more in the end, too! Sometimes just something as simple as listening, and being there for someone else... Is all that it takes, too? Or doing something that is spending just a little bit of time with that person, and showing them you really care about them.

Plus, the better your attitude is? The more likely you will be getting more better results with your seizures, too! Since they can cause you to have so much difficulty with that as well... As many other things, too! It helps you, because you'll be feeling better about yourself also. Plus, it can make things easier for you in the end, too! Since you've got so many issues to deal with having Epilepsy. That you're trying to cope with, and get a handle on inside of your life also? Plus, it'll be a lot easier for your doctor's, too! So, they can help you better also.

I know especially a lot, because I've been there so many times... I've got a lot of understanding about it, and so does my Spouse, too! Since he's had to be there in so many different ways for me, because of it. Plus, so he could let the doctor's know... Things that I couldn't, because I didn't have any memory? Of what's happened to me? When I'd had my seizures, and wasn't aware of what was going on with me either? Plus, there was sometimes those moments when I wasn't able to talk, because of being unconscious? Having to be rushed to the hospital, and not capable of saying anything to anyone. That I really needed somebody else to speak for me instead?

That's just something that sometimes can't be prevented. When dealing with a person who's got Epilepsy? It does often happen, and can be very upsetting, too! Since it's happening to people that others care an awful lot about also, and they don't want... To see anything happen to that person? Trying to make sure that they're ok, but also they'll come out of this... Being better, and get well soon! So, they can go back home, too! Usually if that happens? They're admitted into the hospital, and have to stay a little while; but then can return home. That's the good news!

I know that this happened to me a lot of times, and it was a real pain. I'm glad that somebody was there to help me, but also take care of me, too! I'm also glad that they didn't hold it against me... For things I did? When I'd had my seizures so bad, and didn't remember doing that? Since I was told that I cussed out some people, and didn't have any idea about what I'd done? It's not funny, but it can happen. I also was scared, because when I came, too? I didn't know how I'd gotten there? Or what'd happened to me?

Plus, I had all these needles inside my arms, and machines hooked up to me... That really freaked me out, too! That's what I meant by the attitude thing, but a lot of times... When it comes to people who constantly deal with Epileptics? They know that this can happen, and they don't worry about it. Since they know that this person might not have acted that way... If they'd not had some seizures, and it's caused them to act like that? They're more familiar with how it's going to affect somebody? Than a lot of people, because they're trained to handle it. So, they can usually understand a lot better sometimes, too!

So, I would ask, that you be patient when dealing with people who suffer from Epilepsy? They usually don't mean to act like that, but it does happen sometimes. It's not them really... When they've had seizures, but it's still them? They're just not themselves, and that's what I mean by that? Epilepsy changes and alters, the entire person that has it, too! That's just part of it, and there's not much you can do about that. Except accept it, because that's all you can really do about that other than pray about it all. Asking, God for strength, mercy, healing & coping, with it? That's a big help having him there to lean on, and him helping you get through it also; because I know personally!

Being an Epileptic doesn't just cause attitude problems, but it causes all sorts of problems. I've mentioned a lot of them, too! I hope that it really & truly, helps you... If you've got Epilepsy? If you don't have Epilepsy? I hope that you can help others who do? That you understand, and don't give them a hard time; because of it, too! They don't really deserve that, because it's something that's life threatening!!! I can't emphasize that enough either I don't think, because it's so traumatizing to the entire body. I also believe, that if you're reading this there's a good reason why?

You might not have it, but someone you're close, too! Has got the disease of Epilepsy, and maybe you felt... Like it'd be a good idea reading this, too! Since there's many books about it, but they're not all the same. That's pretty neat, too! I've done this one from me having the disease of Epilepsy, because my Spouse gave me the encouragement... That he felt like it'd be a really cool idea for me to do, too! So, that's why I decided to do this, and share with everyone my very own experiences dealing with Epilepsy? I had no idea... Exactly what all was going to come out inside of it when I got started either?

I just wanted to be honest, and hoped that I can help others by doing this, too! That's the whole reason why I chose to do this, because there's a really good chance? It can help somebody else that's struggling with this disease, too? Of having Epilepsy, but knowing exactly... How they're going to get through it? Or how they're going to deal with it? Sometimes hearing something about things from others... Can really help out a lot when a person is struggling, and having difficulty dealing with a specific problem? When they might not reach out to others, because they're afraid, too? Or maybe to embarrassed to do so also?

I couldn't read any other books about it, because it just upset me, too much! I had to learn how to deal with things inside my life without that, but often there's Movies about it also. I couldn't hardly watch them for a long time, because it really got to me. Upsetting me a lot, too! I couldn't handle it then, but I can now… Since I've been able to learn how to get past things moving forward with my life? It's been a very awkward journey & path, that I've dealt with having my own problems with my Epilepsy. I'm glad that there's a lot more that can be done now, and the correct medications are helping me also. It took a lot of time, patience & frustrating moments, with some awful things happening to me. Before we were able to reach this point, but it's not over; because I've still got seizures that I've to deal with.

Except now I can a lot more than what I've ever been able to before, and that's really wonderful? I've had a whole lot of different kinds of attitudes… That I've also had to overcome dealing with my Epilepsy. Which hasn't always been an easy thing to do, but I've tried to manage them… The best that I could, and when I messed up? I tried to correct my mistakes by making an amends to those I might've said, something to I didn't mean. Or how I acted towards somebody else, too? Having a very bad attitude sometimes after I'd had my episodes & Epileptic Seizures, too? Which generally can often happen to a person who struggles with Epilepsy, too? It's not something we're proud about, but we know how fast it can occur?

Sometimes my attitude was completely terrible, but I wouldn't always be aware of that. Or how I'd acted after my episodes having seizures, and not being aware of what'd happened to me? That caused me to act completely different than what I normally do? Since they can change you so much, and cause you to be a totally different person... When they happen? Making you become unstable, hostile, angry & bitter, too! That's just something sometimes that can happen. It doesn't mean that you're a really mean person, because they can make you appear to be the opposite... Of who you are most the time? That's just part of it that's all, and it's also hard adjusting to that fact, too!

Learning how to maintain your attitude while dealing with Epilepsy? Can be a very aggravating thing to do, but it can be learned... On how to get a grip over your emotions & gain, better control over yourself? When you're fighting having seizures all the time, too? It takes a lot of effort on your part... If you're struggling with this? It also might take a lot of time, but don't give up trying to do it! It's worth it in the end, and you'll be glad that you were able to do it also. Once you've accomplished that, because it'll make you feel a lot better about yourself, too! It'll also give you momentum to do other things that you feel is necessary to do inside your life, and you might have other things you can find to work on, too?

I believe that it's almost like a Rubix Cube, because you've got so many things... That you need to unlock, but also master? In order for you to get the full benefits of your recovery process? Off on a really good track, and there might always be things you've got to fix? I don't know everyone's different, but that's what's good about this also? Not everyone has to deal with all the same issues, and that's great! Since we've got our own separate battles to cope with, but get through... Having Epilepsy & Seizures, is just one of them I know. Doing all those little things that I mentioned before earlier... Will help you a lot with dealing with your attitude, too!

Plus, you've got to have something that you like doing for fun right? That'll also help you, but remember to take care of yourself… Especially since you've got no choice, but to do that. Or you won't be able to do anything that you really want to do? That would make you feel better, and help anyone else either? Or be there for those who love you? That's also important, too! Since it's all about your health taking care of yourself is one of the best things that you can do. Plus, it's not just about your health, because it also affects others around you… Like I've said, before that's so true!

Epilepsy has a major impact on everything & everyone, inside a person's life who's got the disease? That's just how it operates? It also makes other problems harder to handle sometimes, but with everyone's help… Working, together can make a huge difference in the person who has it? That definitely can leave a greater impact than what you might think? Since it helps move the recovery progress forward better, too! That's something sometimes that a lot of people don't understand either, but those around a person having Epilepsy do. The more support a person has with it also helps a lot, too! They need all the support that they can get… When they're trying to overcome this powerful disease of Epilepsy?

That really can make a bigger difference than what you could imagine? It really matters a lot to the person who's struggling with having Epilepsy, too? They might not show it, and try to hide it… Except it really does matter! Sometimes it's easy to put on a mask, because you're afraid to let anyone… Know what's really going on with you? Thinking that they might laugh, and might not understand? Or that they'll be insensitive & uncaring, too? Sometimes there's people like that, but you don't have to hide; because of it. How you're really feeling inside, and what's going on with you?

It's ok to let somebody know how you're doing? How you're really feeling, and you shouldn't be afraid to do so either? Don't let that stop you, or hold you back? You're just as important as anyone else, but you also matter as much as anybody else does, too! So, go ahead and reach out to somebody, because that might be the best thing that you ever did? Just in case you're one of those people... Who believes that you ought to be embarrassed, because you've got Epilepsy? That's not true at all, because a lot of people have it; and more people do understand it now. Than what they used, too? It's something that a lot of people have more information about now, and not as uncommon as what it used to be?

Sometimes it's just those things that can really help you out the most, but don't feel bad. If everyone doesn't treat you the same way? That's not your fault, and not only might you have trouble with your attitude? Others do with theirs, too! So, don't forget that, and everybody has got their moments... When they're in a bad space, but also having a very bad day, too? You're not alone in that one, because you think that you are. That's simply not the case at all, and it's easy to not see that... When you're struggling with Epilepsy? Having a hard time, but fighting the aftereffects of seizures; and how they're making you feel inside?

Chapter 10. Treatment Plans

Everybody has got their very own unique challenge when it comes to this? Coming up with a Treatment Plan… That works out the best for you, and what you're going to use? To treat your seizures & Epilepsy? For you to gain better control over your seizures, and have better results out of your seizure activity? It can be very aggravating, frustrating & dreadful, trying to deal with all of this, too! Since certain things might not work right off the get go, and you'll have to be the doctor's Guinea pig. In order for them to find something that might help you start improving, too? Sometimes that's just the way it is, but it'll get better. I just can't tell you when, because everyone is different; and often has to go through more medications & treatments, than others, too?

Somebody who has Epilepsy often has multiple treatment plans… That their doctor might have to come up with? In order to help them get better? Since things might not get improved or stabilized, in the very beginning… Maybe taking a whole lot more time than others, too! Which can be very detrimental, because it can overwhelm the patient; but the doctor also. Plus, the family of the person who's suffering with having Epilepsy, too? That just happens that way, and there's not much anybody can do about it! You might for instance have one treatment plan that seems like it's right? Except then as time goes on it isn't right, because it gets changed; and you've got to start something new again.

Then that might seem like it's getting better, but when you go to the doctor? You find out differently, and things change once more? Making you feel like you're back at square one again also, because you feel... Like you're starting all over again, but basically you really are. It's just complicated, because you've got to get used to trying to adjust to all the changes? Until something they'll find actually does the trick and works, treating your Epilepsy? Your treatment plan is the most important thing in treating your Epilepsy, too! It's the most crucial part for you to get better, but also help your progress dealing with your seizures. It really matters a lot, too! Especially when you've got to gain better control over your seizures, and how many episodes or sets you're having?

It's also something that's going to vary from patient to patient, because everyone won't be able... To take the same medications for their care, because it might not be what's right for them? So, their doctor may have something else in mind for them, but they'll know... What to do? Since they're trying to help you get well, and have better outcome dealing with your Epilepsy? They'll only want what's best for you, too? Generally most doctor's dealing with this understand what it can do to someone? Plus, the consequences of not having the best care, and needing someone to help them with their condition? Trying to do their best to help others, because they do care. Or they'd probably not be in that field to begin with?

Don't worry if your treatment plan ends up taking more than other people's do? Sometimes that happens, but that doesn't mean that there's no hope. There's always hope of getting better, and having better seizure control. Plus, being seizure free, too! For some patients that happens, but not for everyone I know. Sometimes you've got some patients that have a more complicated situation, too! Having multiple kinds of seizures like me for instance… Which makes it often a lot more complicated, and difficult treating me or them? Since there's multiple types of seizures, too! That can be really frustrating to learn how to treat so many, too?

Let's look at this also… Different medications are going to affect everyone differently, and there's so many kinds of Epileptic Drugs they use for Epilepsy. Some are better for some patients than others, but depending on each individual basis, too! Some people can't take certain medications, because of drug related allergies to the medication. Or their body will not tolerate the medication, too? Sometimes the medication builds up inside a person's system, and they can become immune to it also. When that happens they've got to find something else that'll work, because of the problems that's risen? Plus, there's times when a person can't handle the side-effects of the medicines, too? Not everyone can, and that's the thing… It just happens!

That's why it's best? To let your doctor decide on what treatment plan is best for you? Since they will know what will work, and how to help you the most? Also they'll be aware of all your medical history, because you're in under their care. So, they'll be familiar of any problems you might have? That'd prevent you from taking certain medications, too! That's something else that's also very important in your care, but as far as you getting better. It'll benefit you more, because they can hopefully catch things in enough time… To keep anything bad from happening to you? Sometimes that might not be the case, but try to be patient; because mistakes & accidents, do happen also.

It's also very important to remember, that you're not going to react to the medications… The same way that others might, too! Since that often varies from patient to patient, but sometimes you might have some really good results… Right off the start with a new medication. Than what you'd expected, too? That also depends on how cooperative your body is going to be? Since that's something that you don't never know for sure until after you begin? That is something that tends to leave everyone wondering sometimes, too! Since you've no idea until you see better results, too? You've got to wait it out a lot of times, too!

Sometimes it's the not knowing part? That can be difficult also handling. When you've got Epilepsy? Not being sure if a medication will work? Hoping that it does, and being disappointed, angry, aggravated & upset, when it doesn't? That's just part of being an Epileptic. Sometimes we've a lot more disappointments to face… Than what other people do? Don't let that get you down, because it'll be ok. Things improve sometimes gradually, but over a longer period of time… For some people who suffer with Epilepsy?

We also tend to struggle a lot more with having disappoints, and being able to handle them, too! Since we're suffering with the disease of Epilepsy. That doesn't mean that just, because you're taking your medications… Everything is going to automatically get better right away! It also doesn't mean that it won't improve a little bit, because you're doing what? You're supposed to be doing, and are taking your medications… The way that you were told, too! It is something that you can't take for granted, but you also can't miss your medications either. If you do? You can't double up, and try to make up for the missed dose; because you'll get, too much inside your system.

Which isn't what you're supposed to do? You have to make sure that you stay on track… With what your doctor has told you to do? Taking your medications the way they told you, too! So, that you can get better, and have better results with your seizures, seizure activity & Epilepsy, too! Since you're on the path to doing that… As long as you're following the recommendations that's necessary to help yourself? That sometimes can be the overwhelming part, too! Except you'll do whatever it takes? If you really want to heal, but gain control over your seizures & Epilepsy?

Coming up with the right treatment plan for you… May take longer than it does some, but don't worry if that's so? Since you're not going to be on the same spot as somebody else. Based on individuality, and the kind of needs you have? Will depend on what's going on with you, but your body also? Making things different from other situations, and giving you a different experience, too! That's fine, because we've all got a different experience… When it comes to treating our Epilepsy? Which isn't so bad, and we can still know… What it's like for others who have the disease of Epilepsy, too?

Since you also suffer with having Epilepsy, too! That helps you have more of an understanding, but be more aware… Of what other's are going through? That also have the same disease, and are coping with Epilepsy & Seizures. It also can help you be able to be there to help others who are battling such a difficult thing to overcome, too? Especially when it's not so easy to do, but you can always help someone else? That's struggling with having Epilepsy also. If you're willing to open up, and let them get to know you? Plus, if you're willing to offer that to help somebody else, because you've got to forget about being scared? You have to realize they're probably afraid, too!

When it comes down to it? You've got a lot more in common with them… Than what you might think that you do? Since you've got the same problem that they do, but maybe not all the same side effects of dealing with the medications. Since they might be taking something that's totally the opposite of what you're taking? Being that their treatment plan is a lot different than yours is, too! Just because their medication & treatment plan, is different… Doesn't mean that you can't help them, because you still can! Even if it's a slow, gradual, process that you're both trying to make changes in your lives, together? Dealing with having Epilepsy, but how you're trying to get through it also; and what you're doing to make things easier for you also?

It's something that takes a lot of time, but also a lot of patience… Being willing to make those necessary changes, too! So, that you can start getting better, but also things inside of your life… Have to be monitored, because the doctor needs to see how you're going to do? With your necessary treatment plan, too! Keeping a Seizure Log sometimes can also help, because it's important… To be able to keep a record of your seizure activity, and be able to help your doctor understand more also. Since they're the ones helping you trying to manage your Epilepsy & Seizures, but they also need to know that, too! It's not a bad idea, but sometimes it doesn't help very much either. When it's very difficult to have any recollection of your seizures, and you've got to depend on someone else to tell you?

You can't always depend on that, because they might not be able to see... Or witness all of your seizures either? Making that a lot more difficult to keep track of how many or the frequency of them all? Sometimes that's the case, but don't worry about it... You can only do so much sometimes about certain things, and you'll not always have the control to be able to do anything about other things. That's just the way it is sometimes, but it doesn't make things easier either. It's more stressful, and more aggravating since you can't, too! Take care of what you can? Don't worry about what you can't, because that's about all you can. Besides being an Epileptic you've already got enough on your plate to worry about, and you really don't need to stress yourself out over things you can't fix.

The less stress you've got to deal with... The better off you are, but sometimes that doesn't workout very well either. Since we've all got stress to deal with, but we can learn... How to not let it affect our seizures so much, too? That's something that's a biggie to learn how to do also? Since it's also very important & crucial, for our care, too! The better control we've got over how we handle stress? The better off we'll be also, because it can cause us to become sicker. Plus, we don't want that to happen either! We can end up having more seizures over it, and have more problems if we don't handle stress well?

Your treatment plan should also consist of a healthy diet, too! Since that's another thing that's very important, because everyone needs nutrition. Epileptics needs are different sometimes based off of what they can eat? Without it causing them problems, too! Sometimes having, too many Carbs is a bad idea. Or having very much Sugar? It varies with everyone who has got Epilepsy, because everyone is different. Now there's a diet for people who have Epilepsy? That's called a Keto Diet, but there's lots of issues with that also. Since it can cause more problems with Epileptic Patients, and can be very harmful for them, too!

Some people don't react well to certain things, and that's just the way that it is sometimes. That doesn't mean that it wouldn't help others, but it's not the right thing for me. Is all that I do know, because of problems I have got? So, I just don't use that, because I don't need the extra problems; and have enough that I'm trying to deal with already. It does seem like something that's a pretty good idea... For other people though, but not myself. Another thing is that since everyone's body is designed differently... What works for someone else doesn't necessarily meant that it would for somebody else? That doesn't mean to feel discouraged with things either, because there's still something else that'll help you. Your doctor will know what it is, too!

Sometimes it takes a little bit of experimenting... To find out what's going to work best for you, too? That can be tricky, but it's also worth it. When they find something that'll help get you to feeling a lot better, too? Since that's the main goal, and that's what everyone is trying to accomplish from the beginning, too? It doesn't always happen early on either, but it will happen! Just give it time, but also try to be patient. If you can, because that's really important? You'll be glad that you waited, and gave things a little bit more time. You'll see that I'm right, too!

Especially when you notice that things are definitely getting better, and how good that's making you feel? Since that's what you always wanted anyhow? I know, because I've been there myself. I know what it's like, and how frustrating? Things can be, but also how exhausting they can be? From just trying to find the right stuff to work, and help get your seizures on track. So, that you can gain better seizure control, but are feeling better also. Plus, how unmanageable things can be, and how overwhelming it can be. Making you feel like there's not going to be any hope at all, too! Dealing with a disease like Epilepsy can be exactly like that, but there's always hope!!!

Which should make you feel better just knowing that, because that's something that's going to help you. Having a better attitude, but also with moving forward in your recovery… Dealing with your seizures & Epilepsy, too! Which will really be a remarkable thing… When you reach the point to where they're not happening as frequent? Plus, you're doing better, and have gotten more stability inside of your life, too! That can really make a big difference in a person who's struggling with having Epilepsy, too? It's a pretty good feeling to have, and something worth looking forward, too! If you don't already have that just hang in there, and don't give up? There's lots of things that can be done in order for someone having Epilepsy today to help, but they didn't have before as much medications to use & Scientific Research they've got now.

Which really makes a big difference, too! Since they've got all these things, because that gives them more options… To treat everyone who's suffering with having the disease of Epilepsy? So, that your doctor can better help you, too! Plus, others they are working with also that's got Epilepsy. That matters so much, because it's often difficult treating with the right medications. Plus, they've got to use different ones for each individual based on their needs, too! So, it's important to know that also… Since you're not the only one who's got Epilepsy? Having difficulty treating it, but that there's others like you going through the same thing.

Gives you a feeling to where you don't feel so bad, but you don't like the fact that it's even an issue? It also makes it easier for you now, because there's so many kinds of different treatment options available now, too! Which is a really good thing also, and it helps with getting your care in order. By maintaining the control of the seizures, but also getting better at the same time. Since that's the whole purpose of why you're being treated for Epilepsy? It makes a big difference when things are going at a smoother pace? Than being on the wrong track, and not getting them taken care of the way you need them to be. Since it can be such a struggle getting on the correct medications sometimes, too! You've got to keep in mind that things might not change immediately, and that it may take longer. Since that's sometimes how treating Epilepsy actually is?

That's sometimes the thing that's hard to understand, but knowing that others have it; and are also possibly going through the same thing helps you also. It doesn't make you happy, because they've got it… It makes you feel so not alone, but being on the journey you're going on lighter somewhat? When you know that you're not alone, and that someone else is dealing with it also? It helps you, because you're doing exactly what they are in some ways, too? Which is trying to battle a disease that's difficult to overcome; and not give up hope of your seizures & Epilepsy, getting better, too! It makes you feel not so bad, too! Knowing that you're not the only one who's going through this? That others do know what it's like, and they also understand, too? Also that your doctor might be working with other doctors, because they all do talk, together on coming up with ideas & plans; for patients to help them out also.

Which also can benefit you sometimes, too! Since it might be something that's within your best interest? You never know exactly what ideas sometimes? Your doctor might come up with in order to help you get better? Or how they do either, but that doesn't matter as much as long as they're helping you? That's what they're main purpose is? To help you, but also all their other patients that they're treating, too! Also don't forget to remember… That their Nurse's help out a lot, too! They're just as important as the Doctors are, because they all work, together.

In trying their best to help you, and everyone else that comes inside of their office, too! Which is very important to keep in mind… Whenever you're going to the doctor, too? For the simple reason that you can tell them… What you need, too? In order for them to help you along with your doctor. Which is another thing that's very important, too! Without everyone working, together… On this one you couldn't get the proper help that you need. That's why it's so important, but you've also got an important job to do?

To do your part in helping them be able to help you, too! Since you're the whole reason that you're there to begin with. It's important that you're always very honest with them, too! Since you want the best care you possibly can get? If you're not? They can't help you the way you might need to be treated. Which wouldn't be a very good thing at all either, because if you're wanting to get better? That's not the route to go, and be dishonest with your Doctors & Nurse's. Give them as much information as you can… So, that you can get the help necessary for you to improve, and have a better life also.

Sometimes I feel like a mixed-up bag of marbles, because of what a mess I am. Due to my seizures & Epilepsy, but having to deal with all the problems I have to handle? Now, it looks like I've got another one to deal with, too! That I'm going to have to start taking some new medication for also, but I'm going to have… To do what I did with my journey on Epilepsy? In order to get through it all, too! It looks like I'm going to be starting a new journey, and taking an EPI medication, too! So, I can try to get to feeling better, because I've been very sick for a while; and I'm having trouble eating also. Since I can barely eat half the time, and have trouble keeping it down, too? Plus, I'm just feeling really terrible, and am not well.

It doesn't necessarily mean that I've got Pancreatic Cancer, but I've symptoms of EPI. So, the medication is to treat that, and see if it helps me? To where I'm feeling better? Since they can't get any test results to show up that they really need? In order to help me, but that's something that's been done before… With some other health issues, too! Since the same problem was they weren't having any luck… With getting any test results that they needed to show up, but the medication to treat the problems they were concerned about worked. EPI means my Pancreas isn't digesting food properly, because it's not working correctly for me to be able to do that with my stomach. When I'm trying to eat anything?

With every bit of growth but progress, I've made has came a whole lot more obstacles… For me to deal with, too! Except I'm doing the best that I can to try to do what I can? In order for me to be able to keep moving forward, and not go backwards, too! Since that's not something that I really want to do, because I've come so far; and don't want to go backward. I want to keep trudging down the path I'm on, but hoping that things will improve getting better inside of my life. Knowing that's possible they will, too! With me keeping a positive attitude, and keeping my faith. Just like I've done before, too! Having the support that I need, but also doing things to help myself also.

Since I know how important that is to do? In order for me to get better? I'm going to have to keep doing things that's going to help me, but also what I'm told by my doctors, too? Since that's one of the biggest things that I can do to make things better than what they are? So, I'm feeling better, and I'm healing… Getting through each & every, journey in my own ways of coping & healing, too! Getting stronger, but also keeping up a good attitude about things in my life. Not forgetting all the little things that's so important to remember, and knowing every step of the way… Where I've came from, but what all I've been through that's got me here now? Trusting God, and letting him have control over everything inside of my life along the way, too!

Chapter 11. My Next Steps

The very next steps I'm taking are going to be this… Keeping up my prayers, faith, support, work, journaling & doing all the things I can? So, that I'm feeling better as fast as I can, too! Taking my medications that I need, too! Plus, making sure that I keep all of my doctor appointments, and doing what's necessary? For me to get things under a lot better control than where they are at right now? Since I'm struggling so bad, and having such a difficult time; but I know that I'm going to get through this, too! Since I've always managed to get through everything else, because I just keep going. I don't know why? Except I do know that I can't quit doing all the things that help make me feel better, but also help me live my life feeling better about myself, too!

One thing that is in my plans is this also, and that's to make sure that once I can start eating better? To do so, because I've not been able to eat much. Plus, I'm going to keep a daily journal log just on… How I'm feeling starting my new medicine, because I feel that's important to keep track of? Since I need to monitor everything, and make sure I share it with my doctor's, too! Also so I can take all my problems I'm having afterwards, and make notes… Of any changes that's better, too? Or any changes that's worse, too? I might also have to add a lot of other things into my daily routine of medications. If this new medicine helps me?

I'll need to work closely with my doctor & Nutritionist, too! Since they said, that's something that's also very important, because your diet might need changing. Even though I've had to make a bunch of changes to it already, because it got so bad… That I could barely eat anything? I'm also hoping that my color will get better, because it looks really bad… Since I've been so sick & ill, too! Plus, I want to be able to start doing things that I've not been able, too! Due to all the problems that I've been having, but hopefully they'll start getting better soon! I've just got keep a positive attitude about it all also, and that's going to help me out a lot! My strength has been weak also, but it should get better once I can eat more; because clear liquids really don't do that much.

Especially since I've not been able to eat all that much for a while, and it's been very difficult for me to eat anything? I've had so much trouble with nausea & vomiting, because of all the problems I've been dealing with, too! Plus, I've had severe abdominal pain, but also many other problems… That's been really tiresome, exhausting & aggravating. Since things haven't gotten better, and things have gradually worsened! I'm really looking forward to starting this new medication, because I really just want to feel better. So, I hope that it works, and helps me to feel better… Like my old self again, because I've not felt that way for a while? It's been an awkward experience dealing with all these issues, because of everything I've been put through; but also due to all the tests that's been done without them showing the doctor's the results they needed. Plus, me having surgery, but it didn't seem to matter that much; because my problems continued without my body responding well to the medications for other diagnosis that wasn't the issue.

I imagine that it's going to be another uneasy journey, because everything has been difficult so far for me... Struggling with and handling, the best ways that I can? Except for the fact, that I've done the best I could to do... For me to get through it all, and I've tried to keep a positive attitude. Having faith, trust, beliefs & prayers, all kept but answered, by God, too! Which has really made a big difference inside of my life, because he's been the reason the most... That I've been able to get through the things I've already dealt with. So, I've another battle now, but it's not going to be impossible for me to get through it & manage; because I believe in myself, too! That I can do it, and all things are possible having God inside of your life!!! It's not going to be so unbearable, because it's going to be better than how it's been so far I do believe?

Sometimes going down different roads is a real disaster, but sometimes it's worth it. Since you've no idea... What lies ahead on the other side of that? That might be worth the wait, too! Especially when all things aren't as bad as they seem, but they feel like it at the time? Sometimes that's just how it feels, and that doesn't mean that's how it actually is at all? Since looks can be deceiving, too! Knowing the differences of all things that you're facing, but having all the facts... Definitely helps you when you've all these problems to face? Plus, being able to use all kinds of different tools... To get through them all helps you out a lot also!

What do I mean by tools? I'm talking about all the little methods that you can put, together to help you deal with & manage; these extreme issues, but that's going to help you pick up all the extra pieces you need to get past these obstacles, too! You see I've got my own little toolbox I use all kinds of stuff for, but my toolbox isn't visible… It's something I store things inside of to help me get through all my problems, and it works! Plus, it also helps me, because I know right where everything is at that I need, too! To help me, but some of it isn't materialistic things that I can use? Since God isn't a materialistic object, but he's a person… That can hear, listen, guide, direct & answer prayers. When you've given them to him, and let him have all of your concerns & worries? Or all of your problems that you're coping with & facing, too?

So, just because the impossible seems almost impossible? Doesn't meant that it is at all, and you shouldn't believe that it is either. Nobody can tell you what's going to happen? That they have no idea… About the truth of what that statement actually means, because they're not God? So, you can't always take what they say? To heart and have a final word, because they could be wrong. I know that sometimes there's things said, because that's what they believe? They don't feel like there's any other hope or chance, of survival. However, I don't want to take that for my final choices, because I know they can't predict time?

That doesn't mean that I wouldn't say? To go ahead, and listen to them; because they want you to get your final preparations in order. I believe that's everyone's own choice to do that, but you don't have to do anything… Unless you really want, too? That's totally up to you! It's something they say? Just to give people a heads-up warning message, and that's basically it I think. Since they want people to make sure that they go ahead, but take care of things they feel is necessary to do? Since you might have some unfinished business? That you really should take into consideration, I guess for peace of mind.

There's always things we should do when it comes to others telling us so? It's our decision if we actually do them or not? Since it's our life, but nobody can really force us to do something that we don't want to do... If it's not something that we feel is necessary for us to complete? Before that final time does come, and things aren't going to get better or improve? We've the right to choose what we do? We have the right to make up our own minds, and decide what's going to happen? Hopefully our wishes, concerns & respects, are followed as we so wish? In the end of our life when it's finally over, too? Hopefully, we've done all that we can to make sure we know our heart is right where it needs to be with God also?

Well I'm not sure what the future holds really for me? Except I really hope that I keep getting better, and maybe if my Epilepsy doesn't go away completely? Things will stay stable with my seizures, and I can have something to look forward, too! Plus, maybe the other stuff that I'm going through will also get improved, because that'd help me out a lot also! I know that the only thing going to work... Is having faith, patience, trust in God, but also having the support I need? From those inside my life that really want to see me doing better, too! I know that I still believe in myself on getting better also, and that what I've been through? Has gotten me through a lot already, but having that inner strength has really helped me strive forward also. Keeping that in mind I need to excel more forward, because I still am not finished pursuing the things I want to do in my life.

I also know that a lot of hope has been there to help me... When nothing else was around, too? Except for God, and the support & love, of my Spouse & friends. Plus, that my pets also care a lot about me, too! Since they show an awful lot of emotion... When they realize something isn't ok? With their Mom, too! They know when something is the matter, but they've also gotten very upset about me being sick on multiple occasions, too! Alerting my Spouse, and getting his attention. When I couldn't, because something was wrong with me?

My next, few steps are trying to manage & control; some issues... That seem like they might be EPI, but the medication is going to be new to me. Since I've not taken it before, and we don't know? If this is the problem, but I've been having lots of trouble being able to eat, severe abdominal pain, nausea & vomiting, diarrhea & bloating. Plus, gas & multiple other issues, too! That all go along with it, and it's kept me from doing a lot of things that I've wanted to do. The medication I'm going to be taking is one that is for patients who also have Cystic Fibrosis, too! I've not been diagnosed with that, but I have got Fibromyalgia; and it can cause Cystic Fibrosis also. So, it leaves me wondering if that's a possibility or not? I'm not sure, but what I do know is that this medicine is supposed to be a very good medication; and really should help me?

If that's the problem, and that's what the doctor's haven't been able to find on my tests? That doesn't mean that I don't have that problem just, because it's not been found? I could, because if the medicine helps the doctor said, we'd know that's it! I also don't know if there's a family history of Cystic Fibrosis or not? Or EPI either? There's some things I know about my family history, but not enough sometimes... To help me help the doctor's I see to help me more, because of me leaving home when I did? I haven't got much information that I can give them, but I do know about certain facts that I can share with them. That does help me, too! So, the new medicine that I'm going to be taking is called Zenpep, and I'm going to be taking a total of 40,000 Units daily.

I'm aware after doing a little research about the medicine… That there's a Support Group, but I'm going to skip it. I feel like I'm going to be ok, and that I'll do just fine managing with my problems. Since I've got my own little invisible toolbox of tools I use… To help me cope with all sorts of problems, and that I don't need it. If I start struggling, because things become, too overwhelming for me? Then maybe I will use it, because I know… How hard things can become dealing with things sometimes, and you need that extra outlet of support, too? At least I know there's help there if I need it? I can reach out, and get some, too!

I've got a feeling that's very strong inside my gut right now… Telling me that everything's going to be ok! I'm trying to keep a positive attitude, because I know that I need, too! Plus, it's going to help me more in doing that, because having a negative attitude would only hurt myself. Not letting me be able to get the full benefits of healing that I'm going to need on this new journey. I really need that, too! So, I'm going to do everything that I can, so I feel better, and am back on my feet again… The way I want to be, too! I had a Nurse recently not very long ago tell me that I'm like a mystery… Well honestly I feel like an experiment sometimes still, because of my health issues; but it's not my doctor's fault!

I've got so many issues that are so complex, and it makes it harder to take care of me sometimes. My medical needs exceed some expectations & care, of other doctor's. Due to that being such a high factor, too! It definitely does make a huge difference if you're healthier? Than being so unhealthy, but having so many kinds of multiple issues to deal with all at once, too! That really complicates things a whole lot you see, because they've got much more to deal with. Taking more time, work, patience, but also can be very overwhelming & aggravating. Since it can be so stressful, and also be a big pain… Trying to deal with so much, too! So, my hat's off to all of them who really do help & care!

Since I know what they're going through, because I'm the patient… I've had a hard-enough time dealing with it all, but I also feel for them; because I know that it's not that simple. Dealing with all my health issues too! It's very problematic, and it's a really difficult task. It's not impossible, but takes everyone working, together… In order to give me the very best care that I need, too? So, that I'm feeling better, and doing much better than what I am also. Which is very important to me, my Spouse, them & others, too! Being an Epileptic makes me get very wound up sometimes, too! I can really get upset easily over all this also, but to the point that I'm really frustrated & angry; because it can overwhelm me so much.

I can lose my patience with it also just as easily as anybody else can? Since it's a bigger struggle for me, because of me being an Epileptic. I can become a lot more emotional & fragile, over situations… That others can handle a lot better, too! It can really do a number on you, because of you having Epilepsy. When you've got to deal with a whole ton of problems all at once? It really gets to you, and makes you more emotional & moodier, too! Plus, it can hype you up, too! Causing you to get very hyper, high-strung or bonkers? It can also freak you out, but bring you down letting you hit bottom easy also.

I know that going through all these issues has been a learning lesson… In so, many different ways, because there's been lots of things. I've learned along the way, and have had no choice; but to do so. So, that I could start getting better, because there was many things inside my life that had to change, too! For me to do the things to help myself… That was recommended by some of my doctor's, too! If it hadn't been for that? I wouldn't have gotten to where I am at now? It's taught me a lot of things on how to deal with some of these problems also? Plus, how to do other things to help myself, too?

There's been many different obstacles in my way, but it's only helped me get past it all. Having the tools that I needed to help me, and knowing... How to handle things differently than what I would've before? If I hadn't gathered all these tools from where I'd learned them from? It's helped me to grow in more ways than one, and to have a better life; because of it all, too! It doesn't matter what others think about it all either, because they weren't in my shoes? They don't know what it was like for me, and didn't come from where I did? I'm a miracle, because I'm still alive; and God's been there the whole time for me, too! I know, and God also knows... That's part of the reason why I'm still here?

I'm fortunate & blessed, that I've been able to stay alive. Especially having the particular problems that I've had? That's almost cost me everything? Including my own life before, too! That's something I'm very glad I've still got, too! It means a lot to me to still be around, but also to be able to do the things I want to do. Before anything does happen to me? Maybe I can complete the things I've not gotten finished yet? There's been a lot of things I've done inside my life... To help others, because that's something that meant something to me!

It mattered, and I wanted to do it. There wasn't any other reason, because I felt like it was something that mattered to them, too! It really did matter to them, too! Needless to say those little things really do sometimes... For those who's less fortunate, and you're just trying to help; because you really care? That's something that comes right from the heart, and nowhere else! People do appreciate those little things, but the big things also... That can make a difference in somebody's life, because everyone needs someone sometimes! That's just a fact, and a part of life. We all can use friends that care about us, but that are genuine, true friends, too!

Chapter 12. Moving On

Going forwards I really hope that things will get a lot better…
Than what they are now, because all I've ever wanted? Was for
me to get better, and have some significant improvements. So,
that my life was healthier, but also more meaningful, too! Since
I've had all the struggles that I've had? Going through it all has
been worth it in the long run, but I wish that it'd turned out
differently sometimes. Simply due to the fact, that it was so hard,
mentally & physically; but did a numerous amount of damage…
To my body, too! I know how many times that I just absolutely
felt like giving up, too? Except I couldn't find it within side
myself to do that, because I've always been a fighter!

I couldn't let myself do that, because that's just not me! I'm
not like that, but have the courage inside to keep on moving
forward. No matter how bad things get, and what kind of
situation I'm struggling with trying to get through? Since I
learned survival skills growing up as a young child, and at a very
early age. I believe that's something that also has helped me
along the way with all my battles & demons, too? Everybody has
demons they've got to deal with at some point, and that's not
always an easy thing to overcome them either. Except it can be
done, because I know many other people besides myself that's
done that also! It takes the willingness, effort, change & working
on yourself… In order to do this, too? Plus, being in the area of
your life where you really want to make those changes?

If you don't want things to change? Then the chances of them not getting better... No matter what kinds of problems you're dealing with? They won't! It's pretty much that simple, too! Since you've got to want to have this happen, and do the work that's required for it to make improvements inside of your life? Without that then you won't have the same results that someone else does? Who wants things to get better & improve, inside of their life? That's the truth, but also a cold hard fact! Never become unteachable, because that helps you keep growing; and also to learn more also.

Learning is always something that is a really good thing, and it doesn't matter... What age we are? We can all still learn things no matter how old we keep getting? That's just something that's also pretty neat, because it's something that helps us be more intelligent, wiser, knowledgeable & informed, about things in life, too! Plus, it's a good thing, because we can never learn, too much... That's not going to be good for us, and help us in our daily lives to live as well. There's always things that we can benefit from in life. That can be learned or self-taught, too? Since we can also teach ourselves lots of things that might be important for us to know? Like cooking, cleaning, jobs & etc.

I feel like there's lots of things that are important in life, and learning is just one of those things, too! Especially since I sure didn't want to be dumb? Or ignorant, but I also do have some learning disabilities... That's been there inside my life the whole time, but I've done ok. I am Dyslexic, and I've got slow Reading Comprehension Skills... I was also told I've got Attention Deficit Disorder & ADHD. I've got lots of trouble with my Speech, and have been through Speech Therapy Classes, too! Except it didn't clear up all my problems with my speech, because I'm an Epileptic; but also I've had some Strokes causing my speech to slur at times, too! I've also been told that I've got the mind of a child in many ways, because of trauma that I suffered growing up; but it's ok I'm fine now. I feel at least, because I've moved past it, and have gotten through all of that!

Yes, I've had many people make fun of me, because of these problems… You know what? I don't really care what they think, because they're just really mean people. Who don't understand, and if it had been them going through it? They'd not be making any fun of me at all! It doesn't bother me, because I know that they're just immature, uneducated, ignorant & dumb, for making fun of people who have got disabilities? It's not funny, but they can have their fun, and joke all they want, too! I don't care, because they don't live inside my head; but I don't let them rent space inside my head either! I've learned that other people's opinions don't matter all that much… When you're going through this as long as you've got support from those who do love & care, about you inside your life?

Having that & God, inside your life will help you out more than people acting foolish! Plus, it's a really good way for you to heal also, and do better in your life. There's lots of people that struggle with multiple health issues, disabilities, problems & things, that can really bring lots of pain, distress, agony & frustration, along with lots of sadness. You can cope with it all the best way that will help you, and I hope… That I've mentioned things inside of this Book? That's going to help you, but maybe you haven't really thought about using them before? Now you will give that a try, and see how it goes? That'd be a great idea, because you'll find that it's going to bring you joy in the end! When you pick up a bunch of those things, and decide to use them? Picture inside your mind an empty toolbox, but then stick all those things inside of it; and there's your invisible toolbox of tools I was talking about.

It works it really does, because I've been using my little toolbox for over 18 years now; and I'm so glad that I've got so many things to help me cope with all my struggles, too! I've found that it's the perfect thing for me to have inside my life, because it helps me out so much! Granted I don't have to open it up, and pull out all my tools... That's inside my kit today, because I've been able to grow so much. To the point I don't depend on all of it the way I did before? Which is a pretty good feeling to have about myself, too! Since it also helps make me feel much better knowing that. Before it was almost impossible for me to get through my days without opening up my toolbox, but pulling all my tools out to use daily! Now I don't need it as frequent, because I've learned... How to cope so much better?

That sure does give you a really great feeling inside, too! Especially when you still remember how hard that used to be? Just getting through each & every day? Not knowing if you were going to make it? Or be ok either, because things were so difficult to handle? Having gained experience, faith, trust, peace of mind & serenity, but giving yourself time... Makes a whole World of difference, too! Since that's what it takes, but is so much worth every second of your time... That you put into it, too! You also gain more trust inside yourself when you've been able to overcome those obstacles & demons, that used to cause you so much trouble?

It can be a wonderful thing to do, because it's something that makes your life so much better! It also will make you feel very glad, proud & happy, that you accomplished that, too! Since I know from my own experiences, struggles, battles & demons, that I had to overcome myself. It's all worth every bit of the things you do... In order to get past that all, but don't ever forget where you came from? That's an important reminder, because it helps you to keep that in mind; and not go backwards. Since that's not what you want to do now, because you've started growing in a different direction for the better for yourself? Plus, everyone has got their own journey, story, experiences & battles, they've got to face. That doesn't mean that you can't do it, because you can do anything you set your mind to do! You'll also feel much better once you do, too!

Since it's really something worth fighting for... I do feel like it is, too! Especially since it's all about your own life, and things that should be better. That aren't going so great right now? Except you want them to improve, but maybe you're not sure where to start? So, start by taking care of business with the little things first, and then take it from there? That's not such a bad idea... If you know what I mean? You'll be thanking God for helping you get through it all, too! Plus, you'll thank yourself for doing the work needed to make all those hard changes necessary.

I'm sure that whatever you decide to do? You'll be happy with the outcome. If it's making some positive changes inside of your life? That makes a big difference in how your Epilepsy, but also many other things will be improved, too! Plus, it'll make a difference in how you feel about yourself also. Which is always a good thing... When it comes to improvements that benefit you? You'd rather be optimistic than a pessimistic person wouldn't you? Having your glass full, but not half-full; because then you can't see past the roes colored glasses? Being optimistic means you've got a positive attitude about things, and aren't trying to see all the negatives, too!

It doesn't matter what you do? If you're not making important changes to help yourself? Then you won't have the things improve inside your life… That you were hoping for, because that's almost impossible without some effort on your behalf. It often takes a lot of work on some things, but maybe not as much on other things. Be patient with yourself, others, but also keep in mind… That you're wanting change? So, that's the reason behind what you're doing? For your best interest, and not anyone else's! Everyone else doesn't really matter on you getting better, because you're the patient; but you need their support!!!

So, try not to walk all over them… While you're trying to help yourself get better? That's important, because you don't want to hurt others that matter to you. Or that you want to keep around inside of your life? I know that it means a lot to me to have those people who I want & need, in my life? Especially since they've been there a lot for me, but they also love & care; about me, too! Which means even more when you've got their support? Plus, it's hard on them also when you're going through the battles that you've been facing inside of your life? Since it has a great effect on them, too! It hurts them to see you hurting, too!

Don't ever forget that, because they want to see what's best for you to happen? So, that you're doing better, too! Since they care so much for you, and only want you to be well also. If they didn't? They wouldn't have stuck around, and tried showing you how much they did care? Or put up with all your crap? That maybe you didn't see? You were putting them through either, but you are aware of that now. It's not always easy to see that firsthand, because you're not paying that much attention to it? Except when someone points it out to you or you're improving you notice immediately, and try to stop it from happening anymore?

Having that feeling of self-worth, overpowerment, control & peace of mind... Coming from serenity, but getting it all after you've overcome problems you were facing? Is a great feeling to have, and it also helps build your self-esteem up more, too! Especially when you're dealing with problems like Epilepsy, and you're trying to overcome them? It's something that's not that easy to do, but is something that can be done. That makes you feel much better, and it can make you feel... Like you're on a rollercoaster ride, because of all the ups & downs, that you've got to go through, too! Epilepsy is a big problem to overcome, but there's also other problems... That can go right along with it, and make you have more of a struggle? Dealing with them all at once is overwhelming most of the time, too!

You can take all of your problems one by one, and handle them the same way. So, that you can start getting better control over them all, too! I know simply, because I've been doing that... It's been a rollercoaster ride a lot of the time, but I've managed to get through it. It also hasn't been easy, and it's been quiet frustrating at times so bad! It's caused me many problems with handling my emotions, too! Except I was able to gain control over those also with time, patience, work... It's a matter of progress, but not perfection. Nothing is perfect, and it does take lots of practice gaining control over some of the issues you're facing with Epilepsy; and the other problems it causes, too! That's why it's so important to do things that will help you along your own journey, too?

To me it was worth it all in the end, because I've learned a lot! Plus, I've changed a lot, too! I've also been able to get better, and my Epilepsy is better controlled… With the combination of medications that I'm taking today in my life. That really help me to live better, but also function better… Since I'm not having seizures all the time the way that I did before? Plus, everyone had given up on me getting any better… Except for myself, Spouse, and God, but also some other doctor's that hadn't seen me before. Who were there to help me, and got me on the right doses & combinations, of medications that were what I needed to help me? That's really made the biggest difference in me, and inside my life also dealing with my Epilepsy.

Even though I've still got tons of other multiple health issues to deal with, and some have been triggered… From my having Epilepsy, but also are Neurological related, too? Then there's those extra problems that didn't come from my Epilepsy, but came from things they used… To try to treat it, and caused some issues for me that's not going to ever disappear. Plus, there's those other problems, and I've got to handle them all the same way… One day at a time, and with the same attitude being positive about things improving & getting better, too! Since that's what I really want? Plus, having my faith, trust, beliefs & prayers, in God's hands, too! I also have got my little invisible toolbox handy, too! For when I need to grab my stuff, but use things to help me cope to get through problems I'm having difficulty coping with?

That will also help me get through those very hard times, but also give me the strength I need? In order for me to feel much better, because they've gotten control; and have made me feel so bad? Causing me to feel depressed, sad, glum or overwhelmed? Or maybe they've caused me to have other feelings, and I need help dealing with them also? With God, my toolbox of tools inside my special kit... I can get through all things that try to bring me down, and make my life feel so miserable!!! That's having belief in something that's greater than anything else ever could be, too! I also feel that if you want to really achieve something that you can? Since having Epilepsy often makes that difficult to do, but a lot more challenging... I look forward to those challenges, and doing my best to get through them all!

It can be more encouraging for you, but also give you that extra push. To get through obstacles you're facing, and it doesn't just have to be about you having Epilepsy? It can be anything that tries to get into your way. Everything can be challenging when you've got something like Epilepsy? That you're dealing with all the time on a daily basis. Especially with the way that it affects your life, because it can cause so many problems for you... That you normally wouldn't have? It also can be something that brings you lots of contentment... When you've been able to learn ways to deal with it? Plus, coping with having Epilepsy, too!

Managing all the extra issues that you've got to handle inside of your life, and trying to get to the middle or past that point also? It also can give you great satisfaction, because you've been able to make changes… That you thought maybe were also impossible? Now you know that they weren't though, and that gives you something to smile about, too! Putting a little bit of a sparkle inside your eyes. Also giving you a warm, mushy feeling inside; because you've been able to gain some hope, spiritual triumph & happiness, too! Which even makes it better also, and it also helps you when you've had a setback; because you know… That it's going to be ok, but that this is minor; and you'll get through it like you did before, too! Plus, it's not the end of the World just; because you've had some more seizures? It's just like going with the flow of things, because it happens; and you'll be able to feel better again soon!

All you've got to do is keep your chin up? That'll help get you through it, too! I know from my own experiences, because I'm an Epileptic; but my seizures aren't going to completely disappear. They'll always be a part of my life, and I've come to accept that. Even though I didn't want, too! Others didn't really want, too either! Except now they're down to about 3-4 times a month… Instead of me having them all the time, and having back to back sets. With multiple episodes, but also having some really bad recovery days afterwards? Due to the severe effects of the seizures, too!

It's still hard for me sometimes, but I'm doing better now than before. I'm really glad about that, too! I feel very blessed, because I know that I am, too! It's taken all my life for my Epilepsy to be controlled the way that it is today. It's been a long uphill battle, and something I'm proud to have overcome. It certainly hasn't been a joyride, because of all the other health issues that it's also caused me to have? It's been very problematic my whole life, but since they're doing so much better now… I'm feeling like a more normal person. Instead of a big mess, but I've still got a lot on my plate to deal with. I do what I can?

For me to make sure that I'm staying on track, but also that I keep moving forward! That's why I said, I'm a miracle? I really am, because I've had so many near death experiences? Caused just from my seizures & Epilepsy, all by themselves, too! Which has made me appreciate every day even more… Than what most people might, because I know how short life can be? It can be gone in a split second, and there's no coming back… When that happens? All we have is the time we're given, and that's basically it. So, do what you can to make the most out of it?

You never know when you're not going to be here anymore? Then you won't be able to do anything else again. I don't know… Maybe you've got dreams or something? Of things that you'd want to do before that time comes? If not? Find some, and make them come true! You don't know that you couldn't pull them all off, because nobody does… Unless you try, and find out for yourself? To see what's going to happen?

You've got to make things happen... If you want something to go the way you planned? If you want to have those dreams come true? If you want to achieve something? That's going to make you feel better inside, but also make your life better... At the same time, too! That's having something great take place that nobody would've thought was possible, too! Except good for you, because you showed them? That you're not going to stop living, and keep going down the same road... That everyone thought you were going, too!

You've got something important that you want, and you're not going to be happy until you get it? So, that little feeling of gratitude is what I've got? After I know what all I've been through, but also the accomplishments? That I've had inside of my life that's happened, because of gaining better control over my seizures & Epilepsy. Plus, from the things that I've learned along the way, and the goals that I've set... That I've been able to actually achieve those things. When I didn't even think that it was possible either? After going through everything the way I had for so long? With all kinds of people doubting me, but making me have self-doubt also. Me having gratefulness for everything that's happened, but knowing what could've happened?

Isn't a bad thing, because it's a good thing to have; and know that you mean something! I could write a whole book on gratitude, because I've got so much of it. I know how easy it is to not see? Those things inside your life that really matter, because of everything being so wrong & bad? How easy it is to overlook the fact; you've always got things you can see? That are blessings, and that everyone does, too! It's not something that comes freely, because it usually comes with a whole lot of pain & sorrow. Why? I don't know, but we all have things that we've got to get through... Whether or not it's Epilepsy or whatever it is it all matters?

Chapter 13. My Feelings of Gratitude

I've got so many feelings on gratitude, because I've so much of it! Plus, I know that I'm a miracle, because of all the things that I've been through. That God has really been there to watch over me, and that he's the reason I'm still here. I'm blessed to have my life, Spouse, God, pets, and all the things that matter to me... Inside of my life, but that also includes a lot of things. I've not discussed here inside of this particular Book, too! The reason for that is, because they're inside of another one. An Autobiography that I've done about my life, and things that were very bad... Difficult for me to really get through, and caused me tons of problems, too! I feel that it was important for me to keep it all separated... As much as I possibly could, because my purpose for doing this one was about my journey with my Epilepsy.

Some of it I did discuss here, because it was important factors... That had to do with my seizures & Epilepsy. I've had a very rough life growing up as a child, and it made things more difficult for me; because of me having Epilepsy, too! Dealing with everything that I had to get through, but bringing me down... Such a wonderful journey, and road to recovery of happiness! That's been a blessing in disguise, because it's been something that's given me inner peace, too! Plus, it's also been something that's brought a lot of hope into my life also. My journey dealing with my Epilepsy has done that, and it's done things for me... I never would've dreamed possible, because of being able to get better results from my medications? It's gave me a whole lot of blessings, and things to really be grateful for!!!

There's been so many bad things that's happened inside of my life, but since God was there? It made all of that easier to deal with, and get through… Giving me a whole lot more gratitude, because of that, too! I know without him, and him being in my life? I wouldn't have any gratitude either, because I couldn't… It'd be nearly impossible to do? If he wasn't inside my life? It's made me a better person, but also he's helped me manage things differently. Than what I would've done before, too? Except for those times where I still messed up, and made some terrible mistakes?

That I had to really right my wrongs, but correct my own actions; because I screwed up! Knowing that I had him on my side… Helped me to be humble enough to take care of those things that I needed to fix, too! That was very important also, because he's the reason… For everything that is around, and he's the one who's created all of us, too? Nobody else could ever have such amazing power, and give us all the eternal life… We need to flourish from nothing to someone individually, but grow blossoming like a flower? Making us have free will to do the right things with our lives… Letting us make our own choices, and he's hoping that we do the right thing, too! Giving us our own self decision making, but letting us learn our own lessons as we go?

Which helps give us gratitude when we see how beautiful things really are? How cool, amazing, brilliant & unique, we all are, too? Gratitude is something that we all have, but don't often see it? Why? We overlook things that's in our life we have to be grateful for. Or to be happy about, and if we're not careful? God can take them away, too! When we seem unappreciative? Things can magically vanish with his own doing, because he doesn't like us being like that. He wants us to be glad about all the things we've got inside of our lives, too!

Or he wouldn't have allowed us to have them in the first place? I'm also very grateful, and have lots of gratitude for the fact that I don't feel like I'm cursed anymore, because I'm an Epileptic? That I've been able to find some peace in knowing that it's not so terrible, because I have been able to have some drastic changes. That's caused my life to improve in some ways and areas, too! Which really means a lot to me, because I know how bad having the disease of Epilepsy can make you feel? Plus, I know best how difficult it is dealing with it... Especially when it's so bad? When you're seizures are at their worst, and all you feel like doing is giving up sometimes? I'm glad that I didn't do that, because I would've missed out on some really cool stuff... That's happening in my life, and wouldn't had the opportunity I do with a lot of things now, too?

Right now I've been trying to make up for a lot of lost time, but get things completed... I've been so focused on doing in my life at the current time. Plus, keeping myself as healthy as I possibly can, too! So, that I can continue doing those things that I've got planned for myself in my future also. That way I can stay happy, and give myself some credit... For doing the things that I had originally set out to do. When I was setback, because of my Epilepsy getting so far out of control; and it preventing me from doing that? Today I've begun I brand-new journey, too! That I really hope makes a big difference in a positive way inside of my life, because I really need that to happen! My attitude is good, and I'm thinking positive about everything in front of me; but trying not to stress over the little things I consider really huge!!!

I have also got a Career today, and I owe it all to God, but also my Spouse. My Instructor that I had teach me things to work on, because I needed improvements. Plus, myself being naturally talented, too! I need to make sure that I also give myself some credit, because after all? I've been the one to do all the work! That's a beginning, but a really good one, too! Especially since I've got 8 Books out technically, but 16 total. Since they're considered separate due to them being Paperback & E-book's, too! I'm mentioning this, because it makes me feel very proud! It's all happened since my birthday last year, too!

I couldn't have done this before with my Epilepsy being so bad, and out of control the way it was. Not having the proper medications that I needed to help me get better also, because I was in some really bad shape! It's a blessing, miracle, gracefulness & love, of God, too!!! That has brought me so far along the journey I've been traveling on? So, that I can heal, but be doing so much better now… Than what I ever was before also? Today everything that I've been through has been worth it all, because I'm healing still; but I know that there's challenges I'll always face. That doesn't get me down though, because I believe that it's going to be ok, and that I'll get through it. Just like I've been able to with everything else also! With every little thing that comes my way I'm going to take it with a grain of salt, but deal with it the best way that I can?

Since I know that you've only got to have as much faith as small as a mustard seed, and that's all it takes? Then you can have more, but get through that gaining more hope, too! Especially when you've been able to overcome things that everyone claimed you wouldn't? Except for some reason inside of yourself you found something that kept you going, because that was the inner strength not letting you stop fighting the problems you were facing. Pushing you to move forward, and keep going giving yourself an extra hand… Since you needed that extra help, but also motivating you to succeed. In something that was trying to control you, but also take power over your body, too? That's what Epilepsy often does? It does try to rule your life, and often tries to ruin it, too! Only you can't let it win, and do that; because that's what the disease wants?

You don't have enough time to sit around, and feel sorry for yourself either. It won't help you get better control of your seizures? Plus, it's not going to help you heal either? It's going to prevent you… From doing what's best for yourself, because it's going to make you see all the negative things in front of you. Instead of seeing anything that's a good thing, but that's a positive for you. Plus, it's going to make you have a bad attitude, and not let you focus on what's necessary to get better? You need to have that positive attitude so you can heal, but also so you can do what's necessary? To take care of yourself, and be there for others, too! When they need you to be?

There's not anything about feeling sorry for yourself... That's going to make things improve, and get better for you at all? It's only going to cause you to have more trouble... Feeling more depressed, worse, angry & resentful, because of you doing that, too! It's not good for you to do either, and it's also something that's very easy to do. You've got to get control over that though, because you're the only one who can do that? Plus, while you're feeling sorry for yourself... You're wasting a lot of good times on things getting better for you, but also maybe missing out on some things, too? Plus, you're just getting more seizure activity possibly, because of it? You certainly can't have any gratitude if you're feeling sorry for yourself?

Besides there's better things to do for yourself, and start getting down the path of healing. Than sitting around feeling sorry for yourself, too! I know that's probably the last thing that you want to be doing? If you're struggling & coping, with having a thing like Epilepsy? Especially since it's not so easy to deal with to begin with? It's extremely difficult, rough, and uncomfortable, too! Plus, it's overwhelming, frustrating, but also it's demanding. Due to all the problems that it can cause you to have to handle, too! It's a serious matter that takes a lot of diligence & care, but also hard work... Trying to manage, and get control of things, too!

Also something that's very time consuming, but worth the time necessary... To get improvements that's required to help a person get better, too? Since it's such a problem, but takes constant effort on handling. With multiple doctor's sometimes, too! All of them working, together... Trying to help their patient get better results, and improve so they have a better life, too! It can also be horrifying trying to deal with in the early beginning, too! Since it can really cause some frightening things to happen to someone who has Epilepsy? Worrying others that are often around them, but scaring everyone in general! Including the person who has Epilepsy, too?

Having the best attitude that you can have? Will help you to have some gratitude. With trying to deal & cope, with having Epilepsy, too? It really does work, because I know… From my very own experiences, and things have been so difficult to get through, too! How much of a struggle things can really be, too? Trying to deal with it, and get through it… Needing a lot of support from others in your life also. Since it's something that takes usually a lot of time… For most people whose struggling with having Epilepsy, too?

It's not something that you can usually just get over quickly, but it is something… Requiring lots of patience, because it lasts your whole life? Just if your seizures improve doesn't mean that you're not an Epileptic anymore? It doesn't mean that you don't still have the disease? What it does mean? Is things are getting better for you, and that's something to be really grateful for, too! Anything can happen to anybody, but living with something like this… Is a pretty powerful thing to overcome, and all accomplishments that you have inside of your life that occur? Make you feel very good about yourself, too! Especially when you see so much improvement, but are able to do those things you wanted to do; but were held back some due to you having Epilepsy?

It helps your attitude to improve also, because you've been able to do something? That has made you feel better about yourself, too! So, it really does matter a lot when you can do that? Plus, others notice what you're doing, too? They see it, and recognize that; but give you credit for the things you were able to do. That you wouldn't have been able to do before also? It helps your self-esteem improve, too! Since it has been something you were looking forward to doing? Plus, it opens up doors for other possibilities to take place inside of your life. That might be really good for you, too!

That can bring a smile to your face almost anytime, too! Especially when there's a whole lot of good opportunities that's coming your way? When things have improved, and gotten better for you? So, you've got a lot more choices inside of your life… That gives you a better opportunity for some extra things to occur. Which might be really good for you to have happen also? Besides what's some really neat things happening going to hurt? It couldn't do any harm, because it could help you… While at the same time help others, too! Which to me sounds pretty cool, because you never know what that might be either?

Since you don't know… What God has in store for you? Except it's got to be a lot more than just having a disease called Epilepsy. You probably already know that though, but sometimes you're not sure what it is? He'll show you, but you've got to ask, for him to guide you? After that he'll lead the way as long as you let him be in control. He'll give you the direction, path, instructions, and point you to where you need to go? Then you'll have your answer, but sometimes that answer doesn't always come right away. It takes time, and it's all in his time; because nothing is done in our time ever. That's not how it works for us with anything?

Sometimes I wish it were that simple, too! Only it isn't, and we've got to get used to that fact. If we don't? We're going to be making a big mistake, because we're going to disappointed left & right; about things all the time. That's just the truth, because we need to have faith, patience, belief & trust, in God that he's going to help us… Get through whatever it is we're struggling with, but without it? It's almost impossible to get past any tumbling stone in our way! Pray, pray, pray, and seek his guidance & will? I have a pretty good feeling that you're going to need it. I know that I sure did, because that's what's gotten me through my journey with Epilepsy? Just give it time, because it will work, too!

I also feel very grateful that I've had my loving Spouse… Who's been right here by my side, but has helped me so much! Dealing with all the problems that my seizures & Epilepsy, has caused on us… Giving us all kinds of trouble to get through, but have to deal with, together. Holding on to each other, and not giving up. Was a really hard thing to do, but we managed to draw closer, together. Instead of letting it tear us apart… Like it often tried to do, too! That was something that definitely took a whole lot of strength on his part, and him not giving up on me also. It took a lot of faith, trust, patience & time, but work from him also helping me get better; and having the care I needed to help me do that also.

So, really show those other people… How much they mean to you, because they've been there for you? Helping you along your journey, and on your way to healing. Getting better and improving, your seizures & Epilepsy, too! That they also matter a lot to you. If you haven't already let them know that? Show them that they do, because it's important that they know… How much you appreciated everything they did, and you know it wasn't easy for them either? Especially since it wasn't easy for you at all, too! Give them some credit for helping you, but uplifting you; and being there for you, too!

That's very important, because you didn't probably show that to them before. Dealing with all the problems from your Epilepsy & seizures? Be good to yourself, and be good to them also. That's another thing that is very important, too! They've showed you how much they cared, and supported you? So, do something nice for them, but try to do something… That will pay it forward to others, too! So, it'll make you feel better about yourself. Also it doesn't have to be all about Epilepsy, but you can still do something to help others with that. There's many things that you can do to make yourself feel better, but at the same time you're helping out others, too!